Beating the Odds:

A Story of a woman fighting Bipolar and Kidney failure

By

Saren Keang

Dedication

To two of my aunts who have bipolar disorder like me, thank you for showing immense strength, no matter how many times the psychotic episodes hit you. Watching you fighting through all the episodes gives me the courage to fight this disease with grace and compassion toward myself. This book is the inspiration behind your strengths.

To my mother and my entire family, who took care of me when I was hit with the psychotic episodes, this book is dedicated to you and your care towards me. I would not be here to write this book if it weren't for how well you took care of me and helped me get through the psychosis.

To all the bipolar and kidney patients all over the world, I hope this book helps you feel less alone and that it gives you a reason to fight through life challenges, no matter where you are. I want to dedicate this book to those who have lost the battle to kidney failure and a mental illness. May your next life be free from such health challenges, and may you live a much healthier lifestyle and be much happier.

Acknowledgment

It has been a rather difficult journey thus far, fighting a kidney disease and Bipolar disorder. I have many people to pay gratitude to. First off, I would like to thank the medical team at Guelph Satellite Unit and Grandriver Hospital, including all the nephrologists who have worked with me, as well as the nurses who administer my dialysis treatments. Special thanks go to Dr Friedman and Dr Burk for taking care of me so well over the past two years. I would also like to thank the nurse, Johnathan, for being very kind and gentle during my first fistula poke, preparing me both mentally and physically. I really appreciate that. Thank you, Laura, for always greeting me and smiling during every treatment. Thanks to Maggie, Kim, Grace, Randy, Steph, Yongsook, Jamal, Rebecca, Nate, Auden, and Norine for taking care of me with so much kindness and warmth. My dialysis days were better with your smiles and care. Thank you all.

I would also like to offer my gratitude to the Canadian Mental Health Association (CMHA) team for supporting me since 2021 with Bipolar medications and mental health support. Thank you, Dr Muir, Steph, Karen, Magaen, Anita, and Drew for always having my back. I always know I have someone to call because of you all. Without your help, I would not have been stable until now. Thank you so much.

The person who sacrifices a great deal for me is John R. Alles, to whom I owe the most gratitude. Your selfless generosity in donating one of your kidneys means the world to me. I can never thank you enough. May you be blessed for eternity.

The Facebook support group and the Kitchener Support Group are my other support through thick and thin. Thanks to the admins and the members for always sharing valuable experience and advice related to my health problems. You are my ultimate friends. Thank you.

My emotional support, on the other hand, comes from my spouse, my best friend, and my life-long partner, Ugochukwu Promise Ezeorah. Your hard work cooking for me, washing my hair, taking me to the hospital and dialysis, and your constant encouragement keep me sane and hopeful. You always tell me to cherish life still and never give up. With you by my side, I find hope and positivity. Thank you for everything and for never leaving my side.

Last but not least, I would like to thank my mother and my whole family for reminding me that I still have worth and value, no matter how sick I am. Your love and encouragement help me fight through all the challenges in life. My mother, my caregiver, and my main go-to person when I need someone to share things with, thank you for all that you have done for me, for always putting me first above all else, and for coming to Canada to take care of me when you barely spoke a word of English. To my sister, my nieces and nephews, the desire to still be alive and see you growing has been the fuel to keep me going strong each day and more till now. Your innocent eyes and radiant smiles cheer me up and give me energy to keep fighting. I love you all and thank you for believing in me. This book is for you.

Contents

Preface

I wrote my first book about how unlikely it was for a girl from my background to achieve what I have: two Master's degrees from the USA and travel around the world. Indeed, life was beautiful when I was in America, travelling to over 20 States and cities and giving speeches to many impressive audiences.

However, by March 2018, the fun journey ended. I was returning home to Cambodia, which was great but different. Also, I had two major manic episodes that put me in a pagoda and in the hands of many traditional healers. I struggled to recover. My family almost gave up. People thought I was going crazy and would not return to being "normal". Fortunately, I recovered and was able to work to support my family as before. Soon after, I applied to a PhD program in Canada and was accepted. No one thought I would make it just to be normal, let alone accomplish anything else.

I moved to Canada in September 2021. Life in Canada was met with another manic episode soon after I arrived. I was hospitalized for three weeks, all alone with no one to rely on. I made it back to normal in 2022, and I was doing okay for a year. But life has its many surprises that cannot always be foreseen. It was not enough that I have bipolar disorder; in January 2023, my bloodwork showed a symptom of kidney issues. I took many tests and a biopsy, and by May 2023, I was fully diagnosed with kidney failure. This means that I live with two major health issues, both physical and mental. How I managed to survive and still function as others will be narrated in this book. The support I have received, how I have dealt with stress and challenges, and the ups and downs I have faced will be revealed in these twenty chapters. I hope my life story inspires you not to give up and to embrace positivity. I survive and thrive, to some extent, despite several health challenges; you should too. If there is anything to take away from this book, I hope it is the resilience and courage to fight through life's adversity and challenges to get to where you want to be. May all beings be free from suffering.

Introduction

I was first diagnosed with bipolar disorder and psychotic features back in 2017 when I was doing my Master's degree in the USA. It was my second year at the beginning of Fall, somewhere in October. I was hospitalized for a week. I started this book with the first diagnosis of bipolar disorder. The subsequent episodes, followed by the diagnosis of end-stage renal disease, and life after having these two major diseases. I discussed the struggles I went through, the complications I faced, all the hospital stays, and some tips for how to live life with health challenges. I have a few chapters about the manic episodes, depressive episodes, challenges with my marriage, and the rest about how I have dealt with a kidney failure. I also wrote a chapter about how much time and energy I spent getting the visas for my mother and my then fiancé, and a separate chapter on my trip to Nigeria and the wedding we had there, just to offer some happy memories I built while going through all those health challenges. The narratives are pretty much chronological and constructed mostly from my memories. Some parts of the manic stories were learned from my mother and my family, and those were mostly stories during my second and third psychotic episodes, taking place in Cambodia.

The book has 22 chapters, narrated in the first-person point of view. You may need to read my first book before reading this account, but it is not necessary. It would be helpful, but not a must. The tips for how to live life with a mental health disorder or a chronic illness are all from my own personal experience. I am in no way an expert on this topic. What I shared is just what I learned thus far from my own journey dealing with bipolar disorder and kidney failure. My journey as a patient has not ended. I will have more to say once I have received a transplant, and it will probably be in my next book. This book serves as a reflection pre-transplant and is a testimony that encourages and inspires others not to give up. Suppose I, someone with two major health issues, could overcome the challenges, sufferings, and complications and survive till today. In that case, you too will be able to overcome whatever challenge you are facing in your personal life. May you be strong and successful in your unique journey.

Chapter 1:

Daddy, is that you?

I had just broken up with my ex-fiancé. My roommate, whom I got involved with soon after, was trying to convince me to get over the break-up and move on. The next thing I knew, my mobile bank app received an alert that someone had tried to log in to my account from somewhere else, not my phone. I was panicked immediately. All I could think of was that if the money in my account were all gone, I would be devastated. Who was going to pay for my family's loan? Who was going to pay my rent? How was I going to get food and live in America until the day I had to leave? A million thoughts came to my mind. These thoughts exacerbated my anxiety and panic. When I saw the alert, I was at a public library, 15 minutes away on foot from where I lived. I rushed to the bank, asked the teller to block access to my online account app on my phone, and then headed to one of my most trusted friends, who happened to be good with technology. The immediate thought in my head was that my ex-fiancé was the one attempting to hack my bank account, and since he was the only person who could have known my password, I thought my guess was quite legit. Before that day, he had attempted to hack my Facebook and my Gmail, so why not go that far to steal all my money and make me lose everything? As I feared, he was the one doing all that, so I asked my friend to block him on all platforms and delete my Facebook account completely. I did not want anything to do with him, and that was the best decision I ever made. The deletions of all the pictures and all the memories with him allowed me to move on foot. It was the most toxic relationship I have ever been in in my entire life. I could not be gladder it ended, despite paying a significant price.

After handling the bank report and the account deletion, I returned home to my paramour, seeking to confide my feelings to him. He was not surprised by what happened and told me it was expected. I went to the gym, and when I returned, I felt even more panicked and was losing it. He grabbed me by my shoulders and sat me down on a chair in his room, and he gently slapped my face to wake me up from my panic attack. It was not a violent act or anything like that. It was just an attempt to wake me up from fear and anxiety. He assured me everything was going to be alright. "Saren, hey, Saren, hey!" I was still crying and talking in a panicked mood. That was when he slapped me. I was alert and felt better after that. It was like a wake-up call.

After I calmed down, he walked away from me toward the outside and started making a call in Hebrew to someone I did not know. I was very curious what it was about, but it sounded like an order. It was firm and decisive. I wanted to follow what he was saying, but I did not understand it.

After he went downstairs, I went back to my room on the upper floor and started looking up the history and facts about Israel (where he is from). I learned that it was a monarchy, and my immediate thought was that this confident man must be from royalty. No one could be this confident and wise at such a young age (he was much younger than me).

I heard the door open downstairs, so I went downstairs to talk to him about what I just found out. I demanded that he admit he was the person I thought he was, but he did not. I was starting to lose touch with reality, not knowing it at the time. I grabbed him by the shoulders and shook them, repeating myself for him to admit that he was royalty. He walked back and forth in and out of the room while I followed him, demanding the same order. He decided to lock himself in the room, and I kept knocking for him to answer. When he continued to ignore me, I kicked the door, creating loud noises. I did not care who heard it or that I might have broken the door. All I wanted from him was the answer to whether he was the king or a prince of Israel or not. After about ten minutes, he walked out the door and started heading out to the street. I followed him. He kept walking so fast. I was able to catch up after a while and was pulling his shirt along the street. People on the road were staring at us. I did not care at all. He kept walking for about 15 minutes, then ran so fast to get into a car parked in front of us. Apparently, he called one of his friends to pick him up. I followed the car to a racetrack, but then I lost him.

Soon after, I saw a man walking along the track, and he had a watch on his left arm, like my father. I also noticed he walked like my father when he was alive, a bit unsteady, as my father suffered from arthritis. The immediate thought was that this guy could be my father. "Daddy, is that you?" were my thoughts. I decided to follow him, circling around the track. At first, he was friendly to me. I asked him questions, and he answered. I followed him; he let me. Then I asked him, "Do you need water?" "No," he replied. I then insisted that he should get some. I suddenly felt a caring feeling for this stranger I didn't know before, just because he resembled my dad. I wanted to make sure he got some water and got some rest.

I kept encouraging him to rest and drink water, but he later got annoyed with me and decided to walk home. I followed him to his house, and that was when it all went down. He locked his door. No matter how many times I knocked on the door, he would not open it for me. Then I saw from the window that he was calling somebody. The next thing I knew, there was an ambulance with two police officers (a woman and a man) coming to ask me lots of questions. I stood there in front of the old man's house talking to the police, but I was starting to lose more and more reality. I remember my name and my school name, but that was about it. I was unable to answer the other questions the police asked me. After not getting the answers, and I started to act weird, they finally said they needed to take me to the hospital. I was cooperative for some reasons. They asked me to get inside the ambulance, and I did. I did not protest, try to run, or anything. So far, I am surprised by how obedient I have been with the police.

I got to the hospital, and my throat was so dry. I wanted the water, but they said they could not give it to me yet. They wanted to do some tests on me first. I got more and more thirsty, and all I could think about was that I would die, and I would get to see my dad. It would not be the worst thing in the world if that's the case. "Dad, I will see you soon." That was what was in my mind. I kept laying down in the bed for a while until I decided to ask the nurse to show me the bathroom. When I walked out, I saw many beds with all sorts of patients. The patients smiled at me, some of them bending their heads in respect, so I thought I must be some sort of royalty. I started to think I was a princess. I came back to the room, laying down, and was still thirsty. After what felt like a long time, I thought I would leave this world finally. Then I think I passed out.

The next thing I knew, when I woke up, they brought me to get tested. They did an MRI of my brain to see if there were any impacts caused by drugs or anything like that. Finally, they gave me water after that. I felt alive again. I went back to sleep.

In the morning, I found myself in a different room. One of the nurses told me I am in a mental health psych ward, that I have a condition called Bipolar one. I did not know what all that meant. But I was not refusing the care or wanting to leave. I was cooperative once again. I am not sure why I was. Think about it now, I could have run away or things like that. But I didn't. I still remember being a student at Brandeis and the phone number of my Assistant Dean, Ravi, who was very supportive of my stay in the US. So, I called him to let him know that I was in the hospital, that I could not make it to school for a while. He was very surprised to hear that and said he would invite my friends Kimlay and Thavy to come see me. They did. And I was telling them that I would have to go solve the Palestinian-Israel conflict after I get better. They were laughing. I did not get that. I was dead serious about being the only one who could solve that conflict.

Fast forward, I stayed in the psych ward for a week, taking medication and sharing my stories with the psychiatrist. After a week, I was discharged, and my sense of reality was slowly returning. Ravi came to pick me up and brought me home. He took me to Walgreens to get medicine first before dropping me off at home.

I was not able to talk to the guy/my roommate, the same way I did before. I was all by myself after that incident. I went back to school and wrapped up a few classes. I was okay for about two months until I wasn't. The new challenge hit me hard. Let me tell you what it was.

Chapter 2:

The Dark Period

I was going to school, doing assignments, and doing reading as usual for about a month. Then by December, I started to lose it. I did not understand what I was reading, I could not do the assignment, and I had severe anxiety. I didn't want to eat, I didn't want to shower, and I didn't find anything enjoyable at all. I woke up each day and forced myself to get onto the school bus, feeling very lazy and low on energy. I talked to my therapist, and she said it was the symptoms of depression. I did not know that. I did not have a label for what I was feeling. Without a professional, I would be lost and would just go deep into it without support. I kept pushing myself to continue going to school for a few more days into mid-December. That was when I could not go on anymore. I went to see my therapist again to let her know, and that was when she called the mental health hospital to come get me. I got into the van voluntarily, and I texted Ravi that I was going to the hospital. He was the only person I told.

I got to the hospital, and I started getting treatment. First, it was just medication. Then there was a counselling session with a therapist. There was also an exercise class. There were also classes to encourage positive thinking and increase self-esteem, as well as classes on meditation skills. I do not remember exactly what those classes were called. Initially, those were almost useless. I did not enjoy learning or taking anything away because of my low energy and lack of interest in things. The only thing that was working was the meds. I knew it helped because when I did not take it, I felt worse. I remember reading books in the TV room, and I did not enjoy it at all. And I did not want to talk to anyone or do anything. I just wanted to sleep it off and do nothing.

When I was inside the shower room, I looked at my naked body and felt ashamed because such a hypocrite had touched my body. I felt sorry for myself and just cried. Each shower felt so long.

I stayed in the ward for about a month. I improved after that and was discharged in early January 2018. Ravi was the one to pick me up again and took me to my rented house. I was still struggling emotionally, but I was able to function somehow. I tried to wrap up my thesis and an assignment for one of my classes. By the end of February, I had completed everything. I was shocked myself. I did not think I could do it, but I did. I booked the ticket to return home soon after. By the 1st of March, I flew home to Cambodia, the land where I belong.

Chapter 3:

Water Blessing was my Friend

I returned home to Cambodia soon after I graduated with two Master's degrees on March 2, 2018. I was offered a job at one of my previous workplaces near my home. It is an American school that pays better compared to other workplaces in Cambodia. I was happy because I got to work close to home and was well compensated. Unfortunately, the good and happy life did not last long. In August 2018, a major manic episode hit me hard. It started in Ho Chi Minh City, Vietnam. I went there with a friend from work. During the trip, I missed taking the med, missed sleep, and I drank alcohol – all the things that put me at risk of getting mania. Not surprisingly, a manic episode took place right after. I started feeling drowsy and lost on the way back home, not sure who I was. I slept most of the time in a taxi, so I wasn't causing any drama initially, but by the time I arrived in Phnom Penh, things started to spiral out of control.

At my friend's apartment, I started to think I was good at playing piano. I was playing with so much passion and was lost in my world. Soon after, I had the urge to change into something white because I believed white was sacred. I wore my friend's white dress and then went to the balcony to talk to "people" in heaven. I was struggling to find the words in Khmer as I spoke to my ancestors up in the sky. I was feeling guilty for something. I do not remember what. I just know that I was apologizing a lot. At the moment, I was also thinking I was a princess from a past life. It was all so unreal and overwhelming. My friend was at work, so I was alone in her apartment. I moved stuff from her apartment all over, and I believed that the mini wooden boat she bought from Vietnam had something to do with my origin —that my ancestors had built that boat. I prayed to the boat and was thinking I was enlightened.

I remember texting a guy I was seeing back then that I was achieving "enlightenment", whatever that meant. When my friend returned to her apartment, she was shocked to see how much I had rearranged her stuff. She then asked me to get ready to return to Siem Reap, which was a nice way of kicking me out. She knew I was manic, but she still asked me to leave in that state. I am not blaming her for what happened to me next, but it was a bit insensitive of her. I packed my stuff and went to the bus station with her. I got on the bus, and that's when my head got so messed up.

In the bus, I thought someone was planning to hurt/kill me. The light was off, so it was all dark. I heard someone coughing; I thought that was a sign they were on my team, and the rest were my enemy. I was scared and brave at the same time. I tried to listen to the sound of the coughing and noticed where it was coming from. I maintained my distance from people, and I was checking around myself very often in case somebody was targeting me with a weapon. At the same time, I could not use my phone because my hands were shaking when I held it. I was not sure why, but at that time, I thought the phone was corrupted. I was in a state of fear throughout the journey, without speaking to anyone. I could have called my family to let them know I was in fear, but no, I didn't think of that. I managed to stay calm and made it all the way to the bus stop in Siem Reap. However, that was it. I didn't continue the trip to Puok, my hometown. I spent the night at the bus stop because I didn't trust anyone to take me to my home after arriving.

The mania hit me harder that night. I was not sleeping at all, but I was staring at the plastic tree in the waiting room. I thought I saw a frog that was meant to turn into a human. I thought about the story of the frog and the princess and about life and death. I thought I was reaching nirvana. It was a long, complicated thought, and I stayed awake, thinking about this and that, till morning. Zero sleep. By 6 am the next day, the staff from that bus company arrived to unlock the door and asked me where I was going. I said I was on the bus from Phnom Penh last night, so they asked why I wasn't going home. I did not answer them, but I grabbed my bags and headed to the main street. I was ready to get home then, but I still didn't trust anyone. I walked with three bags and a large painting for about 500 metres until I found a tuk-tuk I trusted. I got on a tuk-tuk and felt a bit less lost. I remembered the address of my home and told the driver so. I made it home without remembering much about how I was feeling/thinking along the way. It went by so fast. When I arrived home, I didn't even know how much to pay him. Apparently, I had bargained with him before getting on his tuk-tuk. Even in my manic state, I still didn't forget my most marketable skill, bargaining. I got home and looked for everyone. I didn't see anyone downstairs, so I got scared. I was thinking a bad thing might have happened to them. I went upstairs and saw my nieces; that was when I felt relieved. I thought I was back to normal then, but things turned out to be the opposite in the next few days.

The last incident at home I could remember was when I told my mom not to step on ants because I believed ants were our ancestors. From there on, I lost the sense of self, and the next thing I knew was finding myself at a pagoda getting water blessing from a monk. The narration from here onward is what I learned from my mother and my sisters. I myself do not remember what I was doing or saying over the next one month. How it went down was not pretty. After I asked my mom not to step on the ants, more weird things happened one by one. One of them was running to the street and jumping in front of big trucks. Then there was slapping one of my nieces for trying to stop me from going to the street. Water was thrown at my mom, my sisters, and my nieces. My mom was the main victim. I heard I threw water at her the most. It was water inside the water bottles, so it hurt badly. I was also talking to the paintings on the wall, and there was much more. My mom believes in a traditional healer. My uncle believes in science and medicine. My older sister, Charet, believes in both. As a result, I got sent to both. My family took me to the Transcultural Psychosocial Organization (TPO) in the capital city, where they prescribed me some antipsychotic medicines to take at home. They did not accept inpatients to stay overnight, so my family brought me back home after getting the medication. They felt the medicines alone would not be enough to help me recover quickly, so they sought other solutions. They took me to a pagoda to get a water blessing. Apparently, the monk who offered the water blessing decided that I should stay in the pagoda for some time to receive treatment. My mom and Charet agreed, and they stayed there to take care of me. They took turns feeding, bathing, and changing me. I was like a baby all over again. I needed help with everything. One thing my mom was most concerned about was that I would not wear clothes or walk around naked like some crazy people she had met before. Fortunately, I was never like that. I even wore more clothes or covered myself up more than before, so that was a relief for mom.

At the pagoda, I only remember the times when I received a water blessing and when I ate lunch or dinner. What else did I do in a day; I have no recollection at all. Then one day, out of nowhere, I was angry with Charet, and I pulled her hair and hit her. I feel bad to this day when I think of that incident. She didn't hurt me back, just defended herself. Charet has put a lot of financial burden on me over the past 10 years, but when I think about how much time and efforts she spent taking care of me in that pagoda and beyond, I do not think I have repaid her back. I also remember liking music. One of my friends and colleagues, Christy, visited me and brought me a small keyboard, which I later enjoyed playing very much. The day when she came to visit, I was not fully aware of who she was. I just knew I knew her. She asked me how I was doing, and I couldn't think of many words to respond. She cried, feeling sad for me. She is one of the people who care about me the most. To see me not in my right mind and stay in a pagoda like that was heartbreaking for her. I showed her the pictures I colored, and then I fell asleep before she left. She wrote me a note telling me to take care of myself, and that was about it, as far as I remember.

Apparently, I was writing letters for myself and others. Another thing I remember doing was predicting which country would go to war. I wrote down a list of countries and told my brother-in-law, Nich, what I expected for their future. I also felt bad about missing out on a conference trip to Malaysia. I got a scholarship to attend a conference in Malaysia in mid-August, but because I was in the pagoda, my family wouldn't let me go. I am surprised I still remember about the trip even when I was not myself. I told brother Nich that I really wish I could go, and he said, "It's okay, sister. Let other people go first. We can always go later in the future. It's never too late." His words were comforting, and I didn't feel so bad about missing out on that trip.

Another thing I remember about being in that pagoda was the beef soup Charet bought for me every evening. It was the most delicious soup I have ever tasted. I loved it so much that I asked Charet to buy it for me every evening around 5 pm. Before she went to buy it, she always asked her 5-year-old daughter to watch me in case I walked out to the street or went to the pond. Monika, my third niece, followed the instructions and always told me to sit still with her in a chair or in my room while we waited for the soup. If I chose to get up and walk anywhere far, she made sure to pull my hand and bring me back. To this day, I am grateful for her protection of me, even at that young age. I appreciate it so much, and I do not tell her enough for that. I repay her by paying for her school fees and school clothes. She, her mom, and my mom were my main guardians. I owe them a lot of gratitude.

The last thing I remember at the pagoda was another patient from Battambang Province. He was having a psychotic episode just like me, but he was violent to the extent that he was tied up most of the time. He beat up his parents and other people, including anyone who tried to heal him. But one thing I still did not understand was how much this boy cared for me. One day, while I was receiving a water blessing, I tripped —out of nowhere, the boy came to hold my hand, which helped me not fall. I could not believe my eyes.

For one thing, I thought he was tied up. Secondly, he was not in my sight when I first got the water blessing. I just did not understand how he moved so quickly to help hold me, or why he was so caring toward me in that state. I never forget that incident and that boy. I heard he was never recovered, and I feel very sad for him. How many Cambodian people experience psychosis and never recover, I wonder. I am blessed to have recovered after over a month. Many are not lucky like me, although, as you will learn later in this chapter, this is not the end of my psychotic episode. I was stable for a bit over a year, and then psychosis and mania hit me again.

Chapter 4:

I was cured by Ta Eisei

(a holy man who has lived in the forest)

In November 2019. I was, once again, manic and lost my sense of self. This time, I kind of knew the cause of the mania. It occurred due to over overexcitement of a new job. I got offered a job that I loved so much. It was a role to work and empower young women of Cambodia to become future leaders. It was something I dreamed about for so long. The offer and the role got me so excited that I couldn't sleep for 5 days in a row. My mind was always thinking and planning what to do next in this role, and I was having racing thoughts the whole time. I realized I needed help when I couldn't sleep again on the 6th day. I packed my clothes and necessary things with me and headed to Siem Reap, where my family was, knowing they were the only ones who could help me. I managed to get home safely before it spiralled out of control. According to my mom, the next day after I got home, I started acting weird again. I became angry at everyone and started throwing water bottles at anyone who came close to me. Seeing that, my family decided to take me to a traditional healer named Mae Thor. After staying there for a night, Mae Thor had expressed concerns to my mom that she could not heal me, that an extremely dark magic possessed me, and that it was beyond her ability to do anything about it. Soon after her talk with my mom, I started acting up more. I went to the street and gave some candies to a kid in exchange for his bike. The kid agreed, and I started riding the bike to the nearby market. At the market, I was speaking only English and throwing DVDs all over the place. My mom followed me and came to stop me from throwing other people's DVDs, but I didn't listen and kept on hitting her. My mom decided to call one of my cousins to help control the situation, and he came to pick me up a few minutes later. When I was brought on a motorbike, I was standing during the whole trip instead of sitting properly. Mom said, "You were so happy and moving energetically while standing. No matter how many times I asked you to sit down, you would not listen." On the way, my mom decided to take me to another cousin's house, not Mae Thor's, because she knew Mae Thor had given up on me. When I got to my cousin's house, I played alone for a while, then, when a tuk-tuk from a meatball seller drove past, I came out onto the street and threw cow dung at them. They were extremely angry and demanded that my mom pay for the damage. It took my mom and my cousin nearly an hour to be able to calm them down and ask them to leave. That night, I ate a whole chicken and started chasing after my cousin-in-law. Then, my cousin decided to take me to one of my aunts' houses nearby, where they hoped I would behave better. On the way, I had a wooden pestle in my hand, and I threatened to hit my cousin if she didn't take me to my aunt's house. My cousin was so scared of me and was shakingly driving the motorbike with lots of fear. My mom was sitting behind me. At the intersection, I jumped off the motorbike, almost making it fall. My mom said I was worried that my cousin would not take me where I wanted to go. Apparently, when I am manic, trust is something I have trouble with. I didn't trust anyone easily when I was manic. My mom tried to convince me to get back on the motorbike, and I did listen to her after a few tries. I got back on the motorbike and went to my aunt's house. My aunt felt so sad seeing me in a psychotic state, so she brought photos from our trip to Bangkok and Yangon one year ago to bring back memories for me in the hope that I would be awakened from the psychosis. To her surprise, I ruined all the photos with a marker, crossing them all over. After seeing that I was still out of control, my mom called my sister to bring me back home. That night,

I threw up sour soup in the toilet, leaving my family starved the whole night. I have hurt my family a great deal, and I feel very guilty to this day. I don't know how I am going to be able to pay them back in this life, especially to my mom.

The next day, my family took me to a different traditional healer nicknamed Strong Grandpa. I stayed for 2.5 days, and he gave up on me because I was disrespecting him. I was always ready to kick him whenever he came close to me. After he gave up on me, my family took me to a famous healer called Ta Ey Sei, which literally means a holy man who has lived in the forest. A neighbor whose son was having the same episode as I recommended that place, as many told her he was extremely effective in healing people like me. Unlike the first time, when Charet was available to help take care of me, this time it was just my mom who took on the role. Charet was taking care of her 6-month-old baby. She had lost her husband to a road accident the month I recovered from the first episode back in 2018, which was September.

My last niece was conceived one month before the accident, making her a daughter who never gets to see her father. Charet was going through a lot. We lost my dad in 2015, and then her husband three years after. It was understandable that she was not available to help look after me again. But all of these meant that the whole responsibility was befallen on my old mom. I had a lot to deal with. I yelled at her and hit her sometimes. She never complained a single word, but was there for me the whole time. I don't know if I can ever repay her back with all that she has done for me. My mom is just the most wonderful mom I've ever met. I don't remember much from this second time, just that I was beaten up by the healer who was supposed to cure me. Apparently, he believed an evil spirit came inside me, and by beating me up with incenses, the spirit would leave my body. I was in a lot of pain, but my own mom was helping the healer to grab hold of me, so who was going to help me? Superstitions are proceeded because there are people like my mom who believe in them wholeheartedly, even when it means their loved ones are getting hurt. I always remember that incident, and after I recovered and went back to live with my boyfriend, I even told him to come beat up the healer as a way to take revenge on him. Of course, that never happened. Besides Mom, my little sister, SereyRath, was the second person who helped watch over me. She was always scared of me, though. She told me later on that when I was manic, my ears were so sharp. I couldn't hear anything she said. She was whispering to my mom, but I still heard her and threatened her to shut up. She had to stop talking in fear that I would hit her. Apparently, I didn't hit her, but I always threaten to. Thus, she was always sneaky when she came to visit me and Mom. If it weren't for Mom, she wouldn't have come to see me, given how much she feared me.

I heard during the first episode that she was hiding under a table or drove the motorbike to the back of the house just to avoid me. I was making a lot of people fearful in those days. I don't know what I can do to repay what my family has put up with me- Mom, Charet, SereyRath, and everyone else. My second sister, Chanroeuy, was also subject to abuses caused by me. I remember another incident where I threw a bottle of water and hit her lateral malleolus severely, and she cried out loudly but was helpless to do anything. She knew I was not myself, so she couldn't hurt me back but kept on crying. My mom was there, and she felt awful for Chanroeuy but couldn't do anything either. So yeah, I hurt my Mom and all my sisters. Could I be any more abusive? How could they put up with me? I owe them a great deal indeed!

It took me around three weeks to feel a little bit more like myself, and I finally left the house of the abusive healer. My mom noticed that I was still manic, so she took me to another traditional healer. This one was not abusive, and he was much older and kinder. We learned about him from another neighbor who saw me misbehaving on the street in front of my home. We stayed there for around three weeks as well. One thing I remember from this place was the son of this healer. I called him 'dad' because he looked so much like my dad. The ways he talked and acted were my dad-like.

I was so happy to see and talk to him. He was very humble and didn't want to accept anything from me. I bought him a soda, and he kept saying "Thank you" over and over. I felt connected to this man in a way I had never felt with anyone else, except my dad. In my mind, I knew he wasn't my real dad, but I wanted him to be. It's not like I thought my dad came back from death, but I wanted to believe there was someone else alive who was like my dad. It was a great experience getting to know this man, and by then I was almost recovered, so it made sense to talk to him. He seemed to like me, too, and I even wanted him to choose my potential husband for me. Long story short, I was in love with him. However, I learned not long after that he moved to another part of the country, so I lost touch with him until now. If I get a chance to go to the healer's house again, I will ask for him. It would be great to see him again and see if I still feel the same about him. I stayed in this second healer's house for around two weeks and slowly recovered to be myself again. I went home toward the end of December 2019.

Not long after, I convinced my mom to go to Phnom Penh with me, telling her I wanted to pick up the rest of my belongings from my rented house. However, that was just my trick. I hadn't known it myself. I thought I did want to stay and live with my family in Siem Reap, but when I got to Phnom Penh and saw my boyfriend, I didn't want to leave. My mom ended up coming back to Siem Reap alone. I stayed on in Phnom Penh with Promise after that. I was still a bit manic, so I caused a few scenes in the city before I fully recovered.

Promise was understanding enough to accept me for who I was and didn't leave me during those hard times. I am always grateful for that. I stayed with Promise in a rented room in Phnom Penh for another year.

By February 2020, I was fully recovered and found myself a job with a marketing research company. Life was okay for a while until I thought I should go back to school for a PhD. I applied to Canada and Australia and got into the University of Guelph in Guelph, Canada. I moved to Canada in 2021 to pursue a PhD. I managed to rise (successful in getting accepted into a Sociology program with a full scholarship) after all those three psychotic episodes and a depressive episode, but my challenges did not end there. Another psychotic episode soon followed my next chapter. More on that is in the following chapter.

Chapter 5:

The first 2 Months in Canada

I landed in Toronto, Canada, on September 2nd, 2021. It was a 30-hour flight, so I was extremely exhausted. My mother had reminded me many times to call her as soon as I got to Canada, but I was too tired to do so. The custom took very long – around 3 hours. Luckily, my ride didn't cancel on me. They waited until I showed up around 9 pm. It was a comfortable van, worth the fee. I was heading to Kitchener to stay there for 2 weeks (quarantine) because I couldn't find affordable accommodation in Guelph for the time I needed.

I got to my Airbnb basement, unpacked some cooked food, ate, took a shower, and then called my mother. She was so excited that I arrived safely. I was glad to see her smile. I then called my then-boyfriend, Promise, and went to bed soon after. The next day, I started getting emails from the University preparing us for the Orientation. There were a lot of sessions to sign up for, and I also had to apply for a Social Insurance Number. The Orientation was hectic. There was so much to cover, and I found the sessions very overwhelming. Over the next few days, I received emails from my professors with the readings for the 9th class. Thus, technically, I only had a week to prepare for the classes. It was daunting.

I ate the food I brought from home and the food I received from two Cambodian ladies, with whom I was going to stay once I get to Guelph. It was mundane: preparing for Orientation, doing the reading, eating, showering, calling family and Promise, and sleeping. I did not go anywhere else during the two weeks I was there. I did get outside to the driveway, sat and drank coffee, but that was about it.

Before I traveled to Canada, I had made contact with a Cambodian student who attended the same University as me and lived in Cambridge (only 20 minutes from Kitchener). He came to visit me with some food and volunteered to take me to Guelph after the two weeks were over. He also took me to get a SIM card and to the University for my first class. It was really kind of him. I offered him a copy of my books as a way to thank him.

On the 16th, I moved to Guelph, and I first met the two ladies who were my landlords. They seemed nice and kind, and I was very happy initially. Things turned out the opposite, not long after. They afterwards showed a lot of restrictions on me and made me feel like I was living in prison. There were so many rules to follow, and the worst part was that they didn't let me go to Toronto to visit my friend, Sumpa. I was frustrated. I came to Canada partly because of her; the thought of not seeing her soon troubled me. In the end, I decided to go see her despite my landlord's disagreement. They even said that if I went to Toronto, they would not let me come back into their house. Off I went after packing all my stuff.

The day I left their house was like another rebirth day for me. I felt free to do the things I wanted. It was like a dream. I wanted to scream out in happiness. I had never felt that free and happy as I did before. I was taking the train and texting Sumpa that I was coming. She was thrilled, and so was I. It took about 1.5 hours for the train to arrive at Union Station in Toronto. I departed the station and took a bus to Sumpa's house. It wasn't hard to find. It was less than 10 stops. Sumpa was waiting at the bus stop when I arrived. I was so happy to see her.

While staying at Sumpa's house, I was also taking classes online. We went to Durga Puja at a few Hindu temples, where I got to wear a saree after a long time. It was fun and memorable. I had a good time at those events. We also went to the beach nearby and took some cool photos. I was enjoying my time there, but at the back of my mind, I knew I had to figure out the living arrangement when I got back to Guelph. I started calling different people, telling them the story, and asking if they had a spare room. The problem was that I didn't know many people yet, and among those I did, no one had a spare room for me. My last option was to call my classmate in Development class to see if I could crash with her. To my surprise, she agreed to let me stay with her until I find a stable place. I was so happy. Now I can enjoy my time with Sumpa fully without worrying about anything. I stayed with Sumpa for about a week, and then she and her husband had to go out of town. That meant I had to leave, too. I packed and left on a Thursday, taking the train as before. I didn't bring much with me — just a backpack with my laptop and a handbag with some clothes.

As I arrived at Guelph Central Station, I put in the address of Laureen's house and started walking there. After less than 10 minutes, I knocked on the door at 92 Neeve Street and found my friend, Laureen. She had a rather small room, but there was still enough space for an air mattress next to her bed. In the first few days, I just slept on a sheet on the floor. Meanwhile, I reached out to another friend who had an air mattress and borrowed it from him. It was much more comfortable than the sheet, thank God. For the next one week or so, I lived with Laureen, managing the small space. She was kind and nice and made me feel at home. Not long after, a manic episode hit me, and I soon found myself in a mental health hospital.

It started with the stress and concern for my family, who were having COVID-19. There were my oldest sister, my younger sister, and one of my nieces who were infected. I didn't understand how that happened since they all had been vaccinated. I started distrusting the Chinese vaccine and started questioning the healthcare system around. I began not being able to sleep and had racing thoughts. Since the vaccine for my family was not working, I started to worry about myself. I decided to go to the Wellness Center at my University to book an appointment for a booster vaccine. I'm not sure if it was the reaction toward the booster or what, but the next day after getting the booster, I had a manic episode.

I went to class and started thinking the lecturer wasn't a good person. I was hoping that he would turn into a frog. I was impatient and disrespectful toward him. I walked out of the class in the middle of the lecture only to find myself not able to open the door. The students in the class started laughing at me. I was furious. I came back and threatened to kill those who laughed at me or any Asian person. The break was soon after, and a student went to report me to the University police, so two officers came and asked me what was going on. They took me to the health center, and then they figured that I needed the help outside, aka a mental health hospital. I went into their truck, which looked like a prison. I felt trapped. After about 15 minutes, we arrived at Homewood Health Center, the mental health hospital in Guelph.

I was feeling lost and overwhelmed. I didn't want to go inside, but one of the police officers forced me in. The second time, the police and I stayed in a secluded room for a long time, and they still had no solution for me. I wanted to go back home, but I wasn't allowed to. After what felt like forever, a young policeman came and assured me that I was safe there. Moments later, a few doctors came to interview me about what had happened, but they couldn't tell me what was going on. The last doctor was finally able to confirm with me that it was a manic episode. Not long after, I was admitted to the hospital. It was the 21st of October 2021, 5 weeks after I got to Canada.

Life at Homewood was something else. It was overwhelming with people of different issues. A few of them like to scream out loud. One of them cried all the time. Some looked really scary with their stern faces. Only a few of them were friendly or nice. I was in a manic state, so I was not fully myself. I was angry most of the time. I was angry with the old ladies who did not want me in their house and let me to be close to the homeless. I was angry with my family for adding so much stress to me that it partially led me to be manic. I was angry with my then fiancé for not understanding my situation. Thus, I was not so nice to other patients. I only said hi to a few of them. I only made sure I got three meals and got enough sleep. Other than that, I did not care much. One thing I appreciated about being manic is the excess energy.

I was always full of strength, and apparently, I was even demonstrating some karate skills (one I learned 12 years ago) to everyone at the centre. One thing I really enjoyed was music. At first, I stayed in the Unit where cellphones were allowed. I was able to play and listen to my music on my phone with the free WIFI provided. However, after about a week, I had an argument with one of the other patients, which led me to be sent to another unit where the rules were stricter. Phones were not allowed in this new unit. The only form of entertainment was a TV, which was shared among all the patients.

There were books, too, so it was not completely bad. It was in this unit that I met my now good friend, Kyle. Kyle had bipolar 1 just like me, and he loved singing. We would sing together during showers (from two different shower rooms), and he would teach me how to pray. He was an extremely wonderful company. We kept in touch even after we left Homewood, and we are still in touch to this day. Life was not all good in this new unit. There was a girl who did not like me and kept irritating me. Eventually, we got into a fight, and then I was sent back to the previous unit. She broke one of my nails, and it was bleeding quite a bit. At the moment, I'm so angry with everyone, and I've been crying all day. It was such a terrible day. I called my fiancé and yelled at him for not understanding what I went through. I called my mom and cried as the pain was quite strong. I thought my life would never get better, as there seemed to be bad people everywhere I went. I did not know how longer I would have to be at Homewood.

Both units had people who hated me. I did not feel safe at either one. I was not sure I was going to find peace back at Unit 1. After the fight, I was back in the first unit where phones were allowed. I liked having my phone with me, so I did not mind being sent back. However, I did not process well there after a few days. I did not want to talk to anyone, including the nurses. One day, I was about to have another fight with another patient, and when the nurse talked to me to find out what was going on, I did not respond. After calling my name a few times and hearing no response, the nurse decided to send me back to Unit 2. I got sent back to the place where the mean girl hurt me. This time, I was advised to avoid her as much as I could. I did as I was instructed, so there was no fight again. However, there were other kinds of tensions.

One day, a male patient in the same unit was angry out of nowhere, and he wanted to hit the other patient who was standing next to me. The nurses were so worried about our safety and pulled me to my room so fast that my finger was slammed in the door. They were looking out for me, so I could not blame them. I realized at that moment that I was fortunate to be manic (going crazy) at a place where proper care was given. If I were to be manic in Cambodia or any other place in Asia, I might end up on the street. Mental health is not a major priority in that part of the World. I could not thank Canada enough for taking care of me during the three weeks I was in a mental hospital.

On November 15th, 2021, I was discharged from Homewood. My doctor asked me how I would get home. I told him I could call an Uber. They usually send discharged patients with their van, but they made an exception for me. I'm not sure why. I was thrilled to be out, even though it would mean I still had to live with Laureen in a small space. I just got enough of the indoor life where I couldn't get fresh air whenever I wanted. I wanted the freedom to walk anywhere, so the same day I was discharged, I went for a walk downtown for nearly an hour. Laureen was happy to see me, but not long after, she started to share the concern that her landlord would not be happy if I didn't have a plan or a date for when I would leave her house. Soon after I was recovered from mania, I had to worry about something else: a roof over my head. The month was filled with new stresses as I searched for a stable place to live. A new chapter in Canada post mania was just as challenging. I was constantly moving from place to place, so in less than a month, I moved to about six houses. It was hectic and stressful. But I fought hard and found a stable place to live by the New Year of 2022. My challenges with life in Canada kind of slowed down for a while, meaning I was able to breathe a little bit. Now it is the time to work on bringing my fiancé to Canada.

Chapter 6:

Remembering a Tragic Moment

My health conditions are not the only problems I have faced in life. Apart from that, I have been through a lot of other things, including some tragic moments. One particular moment that I will never forget was the loss of my beloved father.

After working for two years in my country (after receiving my Bachelor's degree), I decided to go back to school for a Master's Degree. I applied for two of the most well-known scholarships for Cambodian students: the Chevening Scholarship, funded by the UK government, and the Civil Society Leadership Awards (CSLA), funded by the Open Society Foundation (OSF). The Chevening scholarship is for studies in the UK, while CSLA is for studies in various countries, including the US, the UK, Hungary, Latvia, Hong Kong, India, and a few others.

I had to write the applications and give an interview for both of them. To my surprise, I won both scholarships. My family and I were thrilled. The problem was that I didn't know which one to choose. For a girl born and raised in a small village in Cambodia, the chance to choose between Durham University in the UK and Brandeis University in the US was rare. It was hard for many people, especially those in my village, to believe.

I think my application was strong because I was very honest about my background and my achievements. I made sure it was clearly portrayed in my personal statement. I've also been involved in many volunteer activities that show my commitment to improving my community. Additionally, I had super strong recommendations from my professor and colleague. My work experience probably impressed them too, as I worked for international organisations such as BBC Media Action and Family Health International (FHI 360). My GPA was high but not exceptional, so I don't think it was a major factor in my selection. How you express yourself during the interview is also very important. You need to show them your confidence and clear future plans. My advice for those of you who want to apply for these two scholarships would be to read a lot to improve your English, involve yourself in volunteer works, be as honest as possible in your personal statement, cultivate a good relationship with your professor or your boss (so that they'll write you a strong recommendation letter), and project your best self during the interview.

I knew both opportunities were going to be life-changing for me. To help me decide which scholarship I should take, I talked to quite a few people. Ultimately, after many consultations with my former teachers, friends, and family, I decided to accept the OSF's scholarship to study at Brandeis University. The journey ahead was beyond exciting. I was really looking forward to it. However, life showed me the other face. My happy days were met with a major loss.

Two months after I learned I had secured the scholarships, my parents were in a road accident. It was a Saturday, and I should be free. However, my boss asked me to take the 12th-grade girls to buy new shoes. We were on the school bus. We shopped at the Old Market and we got everything we needed after an hour or two. Five minutes out on the road on the way back, I received a call from my brother-in-law telling me the news bluntly, "Saren, Dad and Mom got into an accident. They broke their legs or something." Just like that! Without emotionally preparing me, my brother-in-law just threw the bad news at me so carelessly that I was in so much shock.

I didn't know what to expect, but I definitely didn't think I was going to lose any of my parents. I asked the driver to stop the bus and let me get off near the hospital. My hands were shaking. I didn't know how to feel. I walked so fast toward the hospital. On my right side, I saw my oldest sister and her kids sitting and crying. I looked at a bed near them, and it was my mother lying in pain. Her left leg was broken, and there was so much blood flowing from her left foot. My feet were numb. "Where is dad? I asked." My sister immediately pointed to a room on the left side, and there I saw my father lying and screaming in pain. He looked so pale. So much blood was pouring from his left leg. The doctor wasn't there to treat him. A few minutes after I arrived, the doctor came and told me my father wasn't going to make it. I was furious with him for saying that. Little did I know that he was right.

At 4.15 am on June 29, 2015, I lost one of the most important people in my life - my father. He was my best friend, and losing him was the biggest hit in my life. Fortunately, we still had our mother. Her left leg was broken, but she didn't have other major or internal injuries. She was put in a different room where she had no access to the news about my father. We decided not to tell her about the loss because we were afraid it would complicate her health due to the shock. The funeral of my father took place over two days. My mother had no idea what was going on. When she asked us about our father, we said he was undergoing some surgery and that he was going to be okay. It was very hard to hide from her, but we managed to do it until the last day of the funeral. My mother kept asking how my father was. We kept on lying. It was an extremely emotional moment, yet we couldn't cry because we didn't want our mother to know the truth. The pain was hidden inside, and it was killing me alive. On the last day of the funeral, we thought our mother should know about it so that she could decide to see my father for the last time before his body would be cremated. When we finally decided to tell her, she was in shock. After some moments, she could talk, and we let her decide whether she would want to go to the cremation ceremony. She decided at last that she wouldn't go. She was concerned she wouldn't be able to keep it together if she got to see the cremation. We respected her choice.

My younger sister, Srey Rath, stayed with my mother when I went to the cremation ceremony. I almost missed joining the cremation moment. First, I thought I didn't have to go to the cremation ceremony and just be with my mother. But then, my oldest sister called and said I should come. I took a motor-taxi home and arrived just as the March was starting. I didn't even have a chance to change my clothes (to white ones). I got off the motorbike and joined the March immediately. When the cremation took place, I realized for sure I would never get to see my father's face ever again, and it hit me really hard. I sobbed for hours as I watched the fire take away my father's body.

For the following days, I wasn't feeling what I was supposed to feel. I was sad, but so together that I could hardly believe it. I think I was still in the stage of denial for the time that I was taking care of my mother. I wanted to see my mother getting better more than anything else. I knew that was what my father wanted. Srey Rath and I took turns taking care of my mother. I still went to work because we needed money more than any other before because we had to pay for my mother's medical bills. After I returned from work, Srey Rath would take a little rest, and it was my turn to take care of my mother. Both of us stayed overnight with her at the hospital. Some nights we slept on the floor, and on other nights we had a bed to sleep on. The nurses were all males, and they had a crush on Srey Rath, so they came to check on us more often. That means my mother was treated better compared to other patients because she had a beautiful daughter.

My sponsor organized a Summer program (to prepare us for the rigorous Master's program we were about to take) in Chiang Mai, Thailand, which took place in July. I was pondering for a while whether I should join them. After discussing it with my mother and sisters, I decided to go because my mother was getting much better already. On 14 July 2015, I flew to Chiang Mai. The program lasted for four weeks. I didn't feel like talking to anyone after classes. I completed assignments like everyone else, but my mind was always on my father. I cried every time I got to the shower. I missed my father so badly. I didn't think I would know what it's like to be happy again. Thankfully, I finished the program like others and was ready to head back home in early August.

My mother had already returned home while I was still in Chiang Mai. By the time I returned home, my mother was getting a lot better. I was glad to be back, but the absence of my father was so striking that I was grieving so badly. Because of what happened, I decided to ask my sponsor and Brandeis to delay my studies for a semester. I was supposed to start the program in August 2015, but I delayed it to Spring, January 2016, so I would have more time to be with my family and take care of my mother.

Life has many faces. Despite all I've achieved, I was hit hard by this most unexpected incident. My father was my hero. Despite having arthritis, he still managed to make some money to support our family and provide so much love and care for us, his daughters. His life was far from being called "easy". I miss him dearly every day. My journey away from home would have been more meaningful if he were still here with me. I want so much to share all the positive things in my life with him. I've talked a lot about achieving this or that, but I do want to share that it should not be everything in life. After all, we need people in our lives who truly love and care for us. For those who still have both of their parents, I hope you treasure their presence and give them as much love as you can. My journey after this loss is phenomenal, but it would have been a lot better if I still had my father.

Chapter 7:

Challenges with Visa applications

I was feeling very lonely, so I was thinking I could bring both my mom and Promise to Canada. I was working on both visas. Mom's visa was straightforward. I was not under much stress working on her visa. And as it should be, I got approval without any issue, although it took 11 months to hear back from the IRCC. Promise's visa, on the other hand, was complicated, and it took a lot from me to complete it. The first time around, I did not have anyone to help me. I was working on it all by myself, without any guidance, and I expected to be rejected. This time, I knew I needed to find some guidance to help me reapply.

During my PhD studies, I knew a friend from Nigeria who successfully brought his wife to Canada. I got in touch with him and asked for advice on preparing the application. He guided me throughout, and one of the supporting documents he recommended for my application was an explanation letter. In my first application, I did not submit this letter. This second time around, I worked on that letter. I included so much information, including my acceptance letter, my scholarship letter, my degrees, Promise's degree, my transcript, my birth certificate, my study permit, my student ID, and a copy of my passport, as well as Promise's bank statement. We submitted all that information and proof of living together, but we still failed.

On the day I received the email and the notification that the application had been rejected, I almost cried. I was working very hard on it, and it still wasn't approved. I did not know what else I could do. I immediately headed to the friend who had given me advice to ask how else I could get approval. He and his wife comforted me, brought me Nigerian food, and I felt better. But initially, I almost cried in front of them. I was very stressed. They advised me to get married to my husband, so there is stronger evidence of our relationship. They also advised adding a few more supporting documents to strengthen the application. They were comforting me with this and that, and after a while, I was able to calm down. I did not cry, but I felt very discouraged and sad. The next thing I knew, I needed to book a flight ticket and head to Nigeria. The storm of stress and mental health challenges was about to be met with some positive changes and happy moments.

Chapter 8:

The Rainbows After the Storms

Since we failed to get the visa for Promise two times on a row, our last resort was to get married and submit the marriage certificate as proof of relationship. It was my fourth semester when I decided to go to Nigeria and get married. The idea to go there came up at the last minute. I had already started the classes and thought it wouldn't make sense to leave in the middle of them, so I looked up the flight cost for the month after, which was October. Seeing that the cost was affordable in that month, I decided to get ready then. There I was, booking the ticket on October 1st from Toronto to Abuja, Nigeria, with a transit in Frankfurt, Germany.

The trip was pleasant, neither too long nor too short. I had a nice breakfast at Frankfurt Airport. Their coffee smelled extremely good, and their croissant was delicious. They accepted my Canadian debit card, so that was convenient. I waited at the airport for about 4 hours before heading to Abuja. Promise had arranged for an immigration man to receive me at the airport. He was supposed to arrange my visa and everything else, so I shouldn't have been worried about anything. However, it didn't take away my worries. I was scared that he wouldn't show up, and I would be lost in the airport alone. In my mind, I kept praying that I would see him right away when I arrived at the Abuja airport. Thankfully, my prayer was answered. As I landed at the airport and walked into immigration, I saw the man waiting, smiling happily when he saw me. He said hi and asked me to follow him to a room where officers were handling visas for foreign travellers. We waited about 10 minutes, and then I got called to take a picture for the visa. A few minutes later, I got my visa, and we headed out of the international area of the airport. It was already around 8 pm, so there were no flights to Delta State at that time. We managed to buy a ticket for Delta State the next day and then checked into a hotel. It was about 15 minutes away from the airport. The hotel was decent, but there was no light in the bathroom. I told the manager, and it took them almost an hour to get a repairman to fix the light. There were dinners at the hotel, but we didn't like the food, so the immigration officer went out to get us additional meals. It was rice and fish. I enjoyed it. After dinner, the immigration man took off to his house and told me he'd be back in the morning to take me to the airport. There was no Wi-Fi, but my phone plan had data for international calls, so I used it, only to regret it later because it was so expensive. I called Promise and let him know I was safe and sound before I went to bed.

I slept well and woke up around 6 am. I took a shower, rearranged my clothes in the luggage, and waited for the Immigration man. He arrived around 7 am and took me to the airport right away. On the way, we saw men armed with AK-47s guarding the street. They must take security very seriously, but for me, someone coming from a country where we rarely see guns, I was alarmed and scared a little bit. We arrived at the airport soon after, and I exchanged some money for my trip in case I wanted to buy food. Indeed, it was helpful later on because I did feel hungry. The immigration man assisted me with checking in and ensuring my luggage was properly tagged, and he walked me past security to the boarding room. Once we arrived at my gate, he said he needed to leave. I was sure I could take care of myself from there onward, so I let him go. I gave him some money as a thank-you, and he smiled and left. I was hungry, and my flight wasn't ready for another hour. I decided to grab a bit to eat, and I spent around 7 USD on a plate of rice and chicken and a piece of snack

An hour later, which was around 9 am, I flew out to Delta State. My excitement spiked. I was beyond happy and thrilled to see my fiancé after 13 months apart. I was counting the minutes in my head and checking the time on my phone. The flight was 1 hour and 10 minutes, but it felt like forever because I wanted to see my fiancé so badly. When I arrived in Asaba, the capital city of Delta State, I called Promise immediately, only to learn that he was still on the way. I was a bit disappointed because I was expecting to see him right away. I waited outside for about 10 minutes, and he arrived. I could barely recognize the man I fell in love with. He looked different from when I last saw him.

I'm not sure exactly what, but it was still him, of course. He kissed me on the lips briefly and then took my luggage and started walking to the car. I followed him to the car and met two of his friends who joined him on the trip to pick me up. It was a 45-minute drive from Promise's house to the airport and vice versa. I was proud to see Promise driving so skillfully. He played loud music in the car and sang along happily. I was smiling all the way as I got to sit next to him and see him being so happy. Forty-five minutes later, we arrived at his house. It was a nice and beautiful house. Promise built the house with his own income from working in Cambodia. I was extremely proud of him. Later next week, when we were coming back from the market, Promise asked me, "Whose house is this?" I said, "Yours." He immediately responded: "No, it's ours." I was smiling inside, filled with happiness as I thought he was extremely sweet.

I arrived at Promise's house on the 3rd of October, and Promise's birthday was on the 4th. We celebrated by cooking a whole ram and invited around 20 friends. That was my first time eating ram meat, and I enjoyed it immensely. However, my teeth ached soon after eating too much meat. It was so unfortunate to have a toothache as I missed out on a lot of delicious food. It took me a few days to get rid of the pain and be able to eat anything I wanted.

I was still working as a Teaching Assistant and Research Assistant while in Nigeria, so the trip wasn't just relaxing and fun. Work was involved. There was no Wi-Fi at Promise's house, but we used the phone's hotspot. The internet speed was decent. I was able to check emails, research, and analyzed data. Promise took me out to his friends' house or to eat at different places. All the foods were amazing, and his friends were all nice to me. I was enjoying myself a great deal. On the 13th of October, we went to the Marriage Minister to get married. I dressed up in a white gown, and Promise put on a blazer. We signed the marriage certificate and took photos. There wasn't a ceremony; it was just the official gathering and signing. I didn't mind about that. I love him, and we didn't have much money. We couldn't afford a big ceremony then, but we promised each other that we would have a nice ceremony in Cambodia a few years later.

I continued to grade papers and researched as time went by, while going out with Promise to eat and party. I had three weeks with Promise, and it went by so fast. My last memorable trip was when I went to a local market with him to buy food for my friends back in Canada. I took a lot of photos of a variety of food being displayed for sale in that market. Some of the pictures are included below in this chapter.

Overall, my trip was amazing. It was so great to reunite with Promise, see his dad, sister, and friends, and witness the lives of Nigerians. Traveling is always rewarding. This part of my journey probably doesn't fall under the surviving theme. It was more of thriving. But I had to include this chapter to provide a full picture of my life post-disaster and before a new challenge. I returned to Canada on the 22nd of October and resumed life as a PhD student. That didn't last long, unfortunately. Follow more for what went down that ended my PhD journey.

Some of my wedding pictures

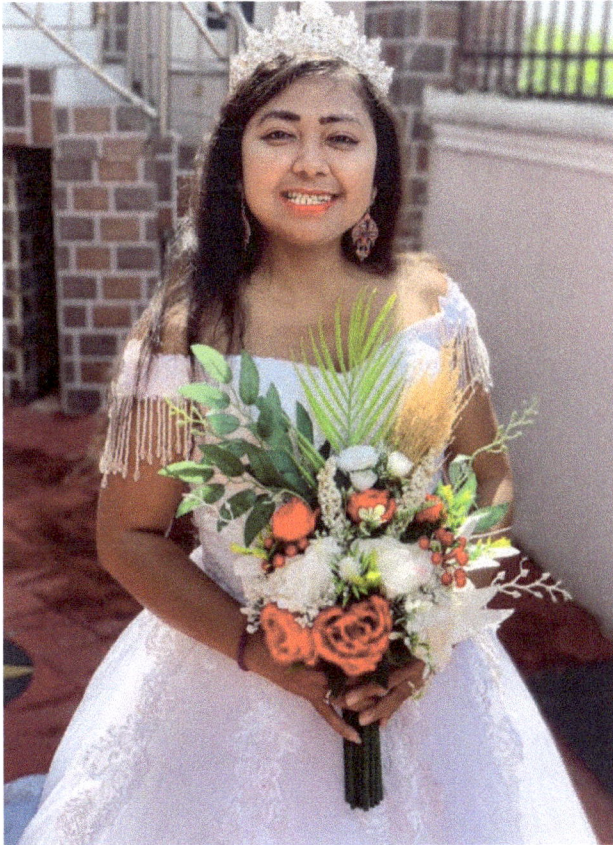

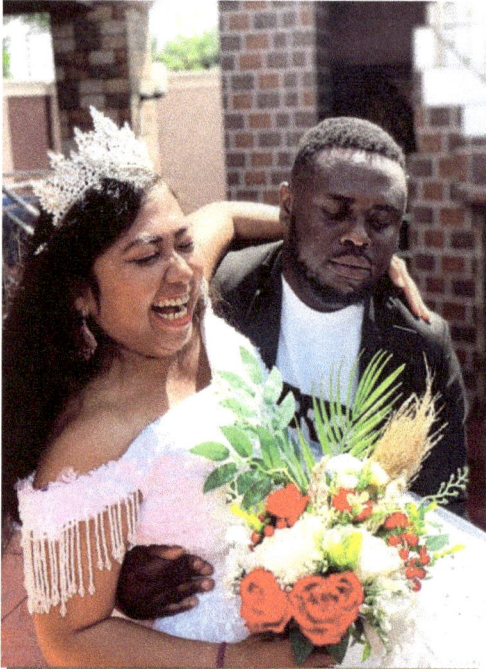

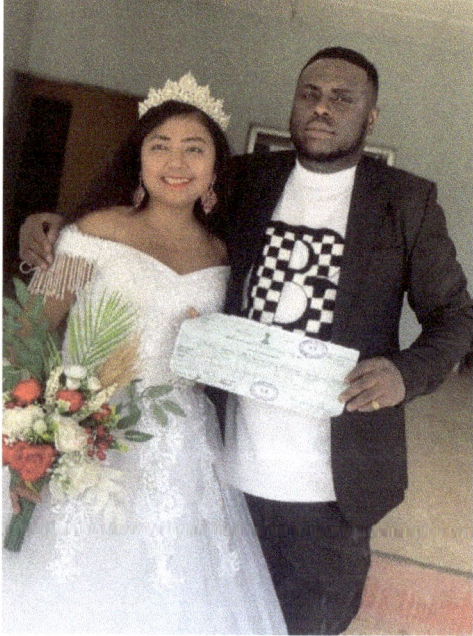

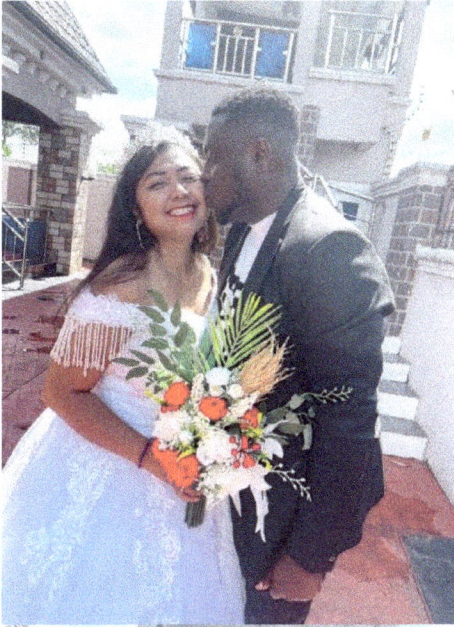
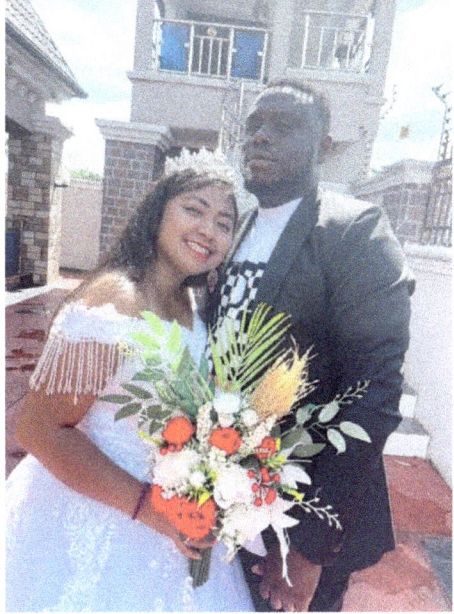

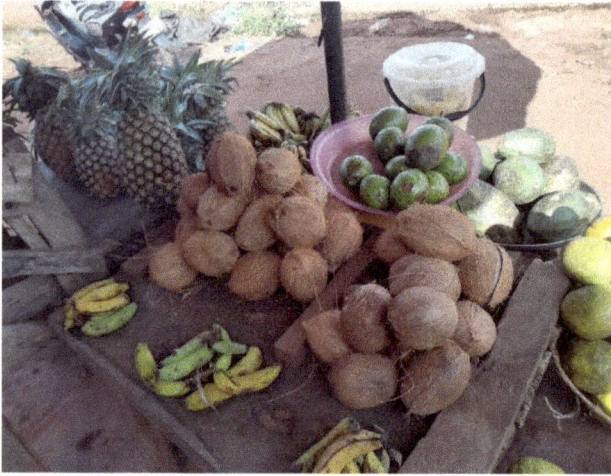

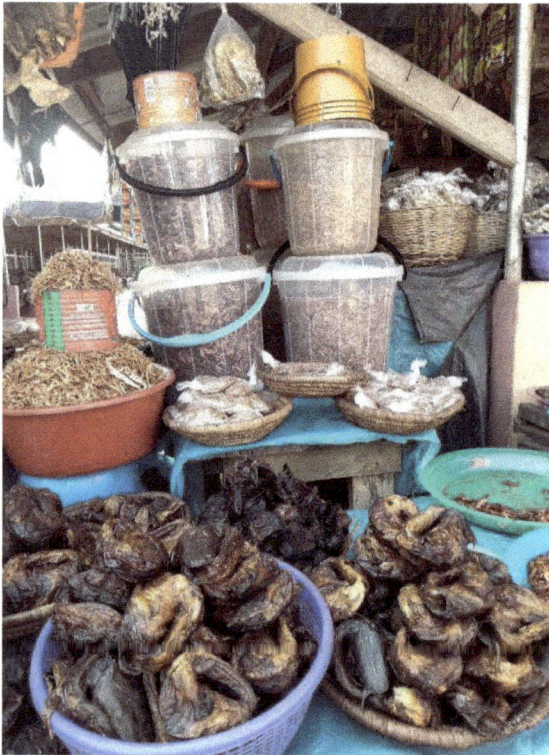

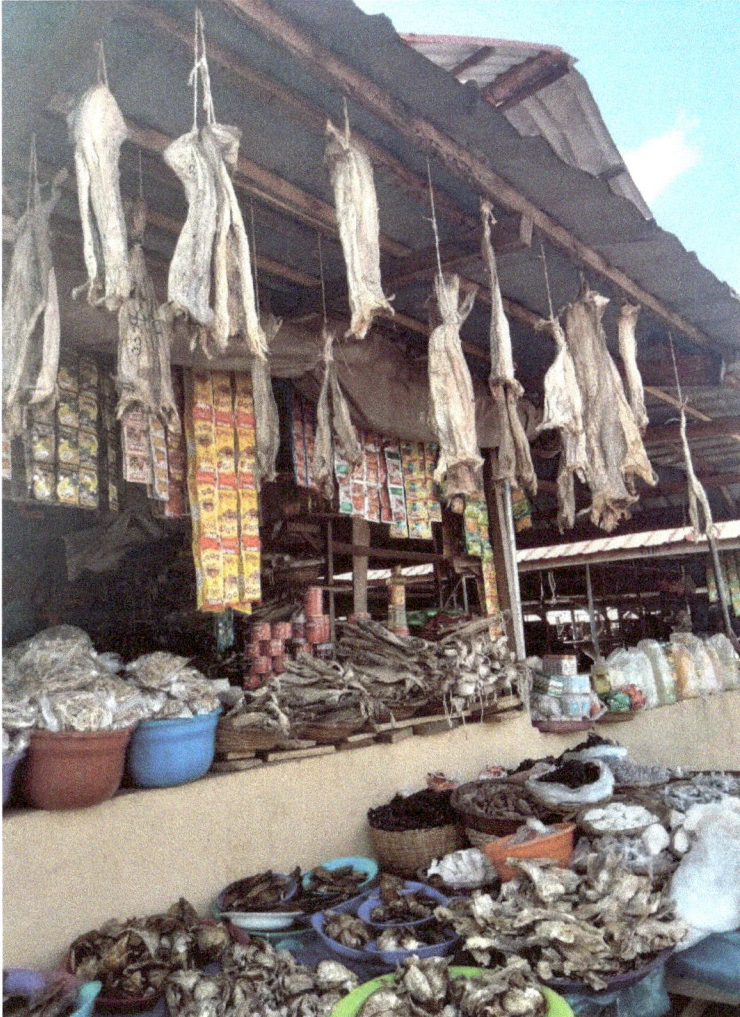

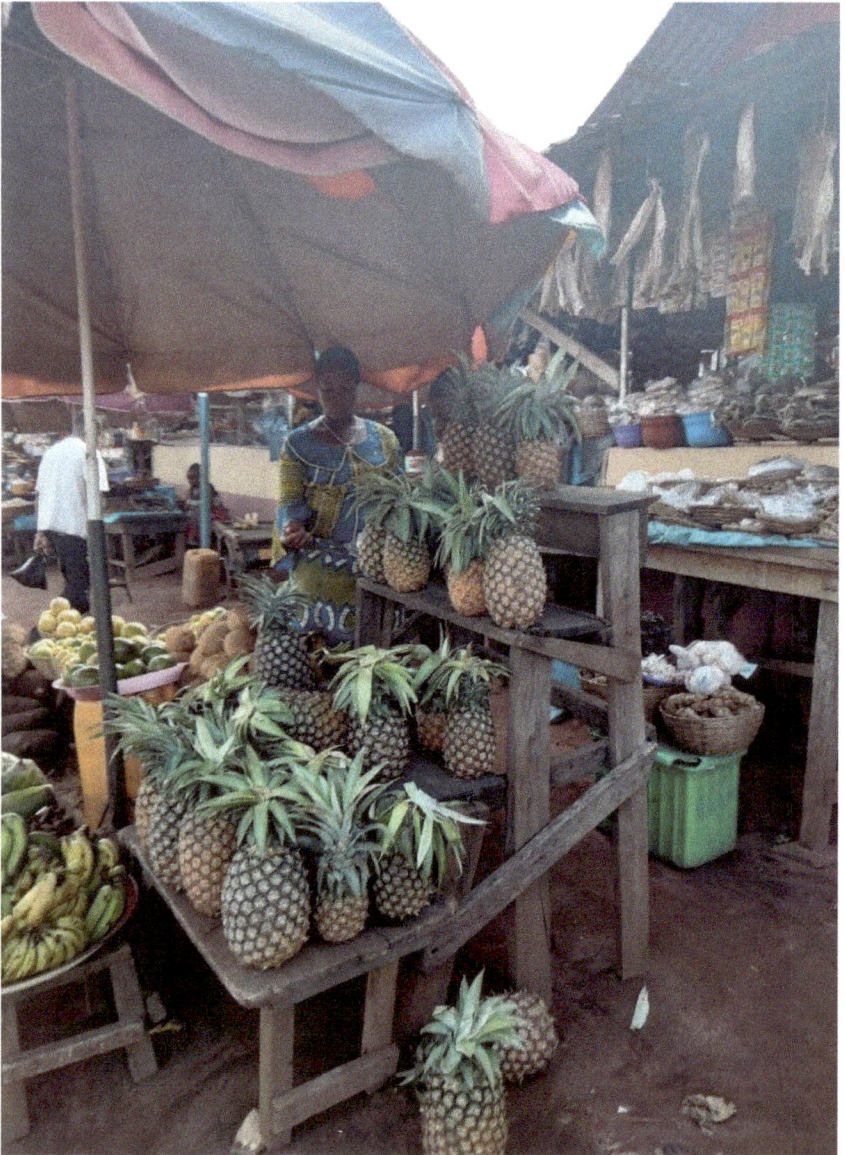

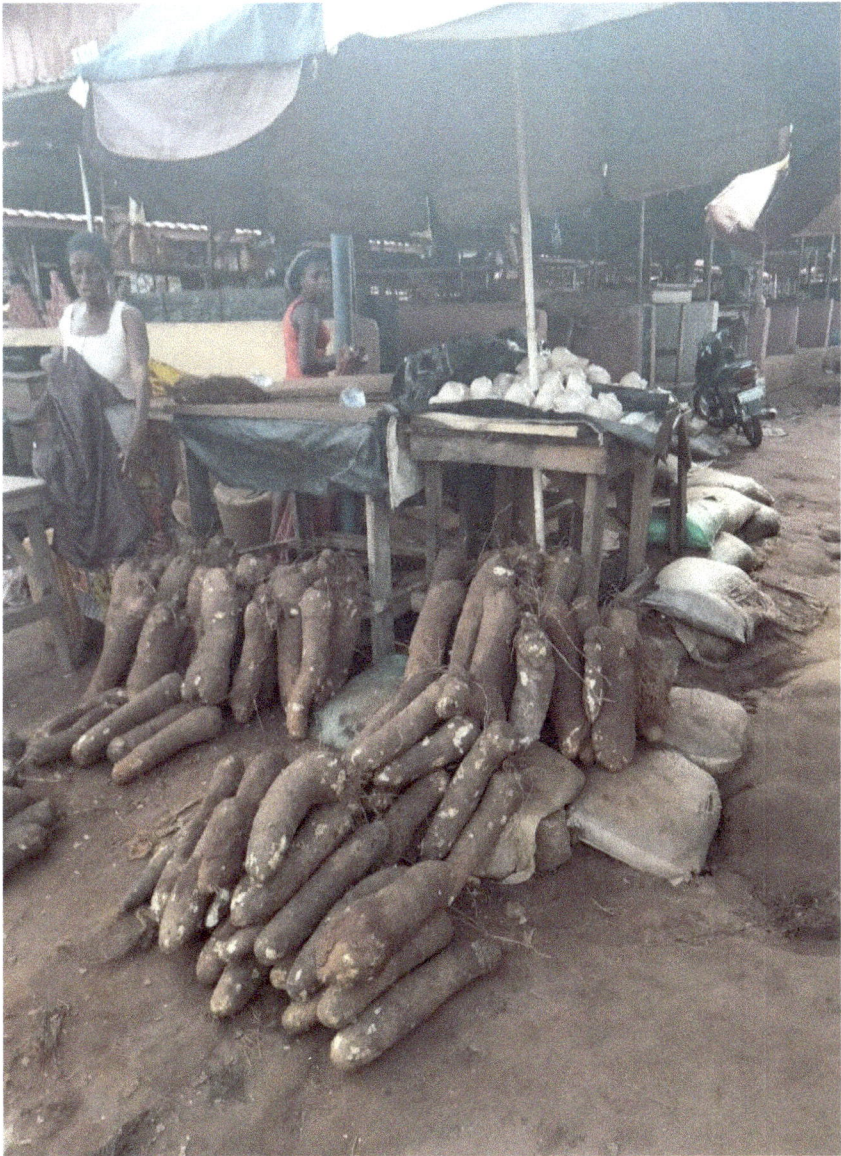

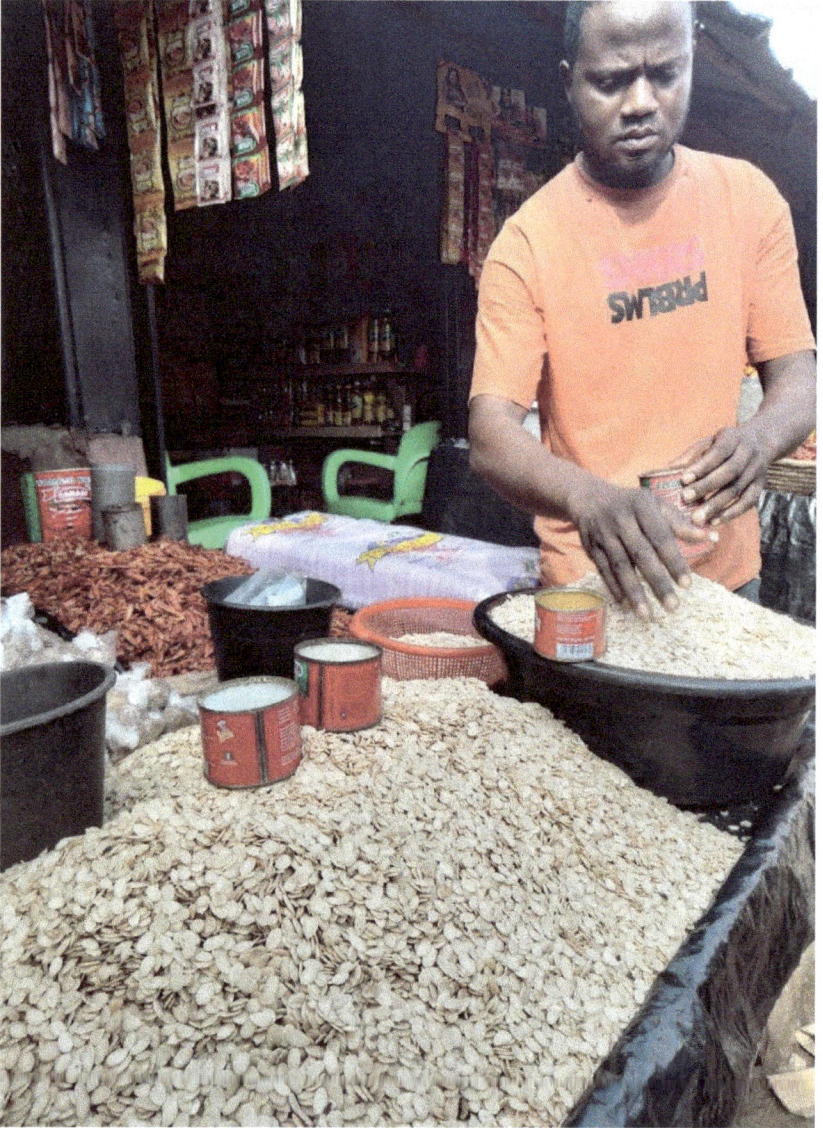

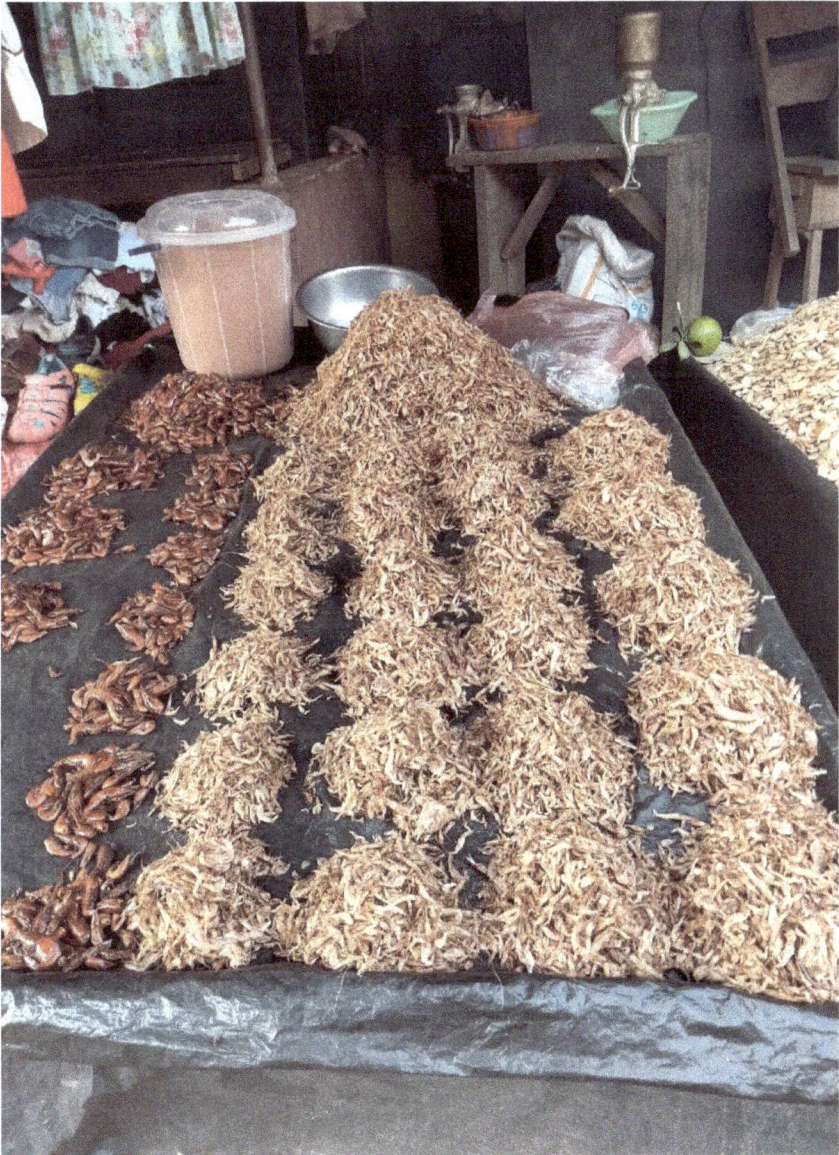

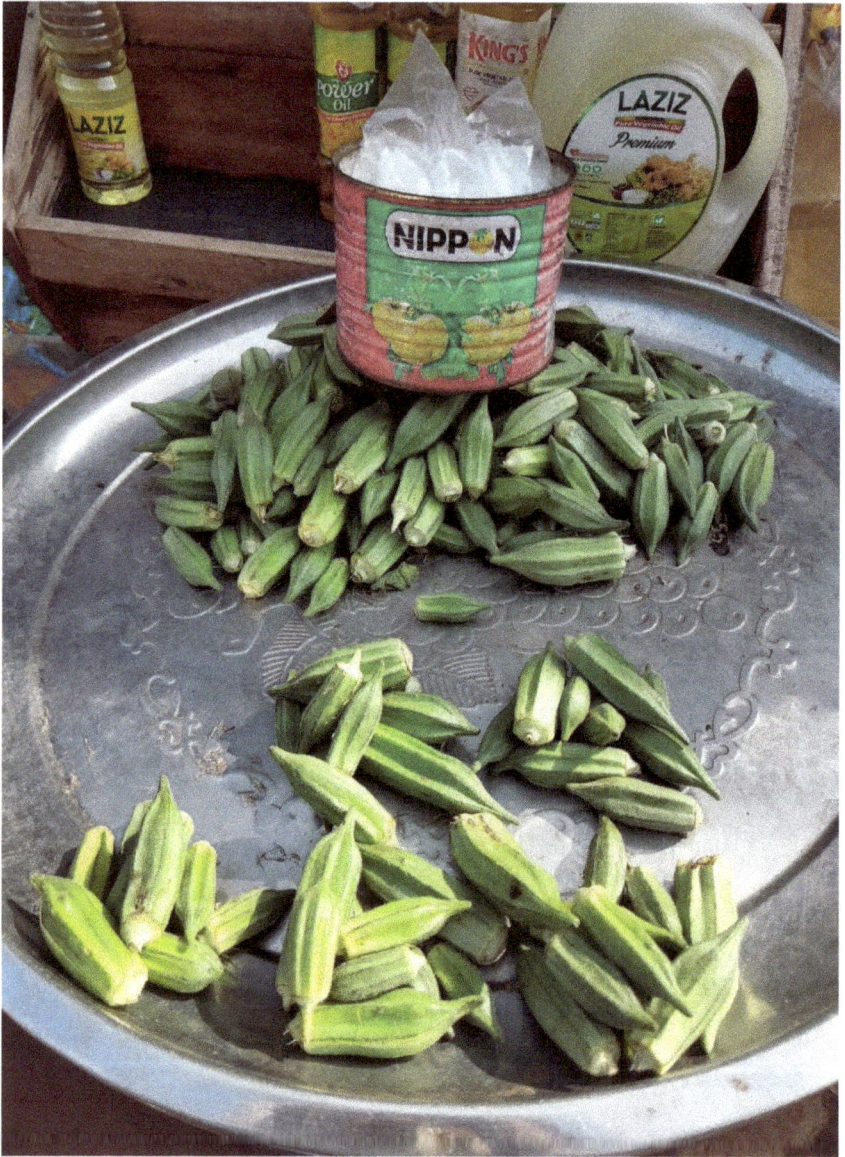

Chapter 9:

Classes and Medical Appointments

My mother finally got the visa approval in November 2022. She doesn't speak any English and isn't able to navigate the airport, so we asked around if anyone was travelling to Canada around December or early 2023. Fortunately, a daughter of one of my mom's friends was coming to visit from Canada and was returning in January 2023. My mother was thrilled to hear that and decided to tag along with that young woman.

A little before I went to Nigeria, and while I was in Nigeria, I started having strange symptoms of extensive sleepiness and tiredness that I had never experienced before. Therefore, when I returned home from Nigeria, I decided to have my blood tested at a local lab in Guelph. The first blood work showed an elevated creatinine level, but it was not concerning. My family doctor had informed me that something was not right, but he had not warned me yet. In early January, right before my mother arrived, I was asked to have my blood checked one more time to monitor the creatinine level. My mother arrived on January 17. The next day, the 18th, I got a call from my family doctor's office that I needed to go to the Emergency Room at the Guelph General Hospital because my blood work showed a serious concern. I was shocked by the news and started to worry. I told my mother I had to go to the Emergency room, and she was scared hearing that. She just arrived a day ago, and that's what happened? I felt sad about leaving her alone in my room just one day after she arrived, but I had no choice. I called an Uber and headed to the ER around 10 am in the morning.

When I got to the hospital, I told them my family doctor sent me because of concerns about my blood work, so they wanted to confirm the results by having me repeat the blood work. I waited for the blood work result for a few hours, and when the doctor was ready to talk to me, they said my kidney was failing. My creatine level was higher than a regular level, and I will need to see a kidney specialist, known as a nephrologist. But the appointment was not until April. However, they did have a biopsy appointment for me in March to find out the cause of my kidney failure before I got to see the nephrologist. I was in shock when I heard the news, but I did not get too sad. I did not comprehend how serious that was. I was asked to return home and wait to see the nephrologist for the next step, since they had already made an appointment for me. I went home and told my mother what the doctor said, and she was shocked. That was not something she expected upon her arrival. She was just a bit happy to see me after over a year of being part of it, and then boom —the bad news. As a mother, there is nothing else more saddening than hearing that your child is sick. My mother looked very worried, but I tried to console her, assuring her I would be okay.

After that visit to the ER, my family doctor had asked me to have my blood checked every two weeks. I would go to class, and then go to the life lab biweekly. The life lab was in Guelph, so arranging transportation was not hard. I just had to take a bus from my home, and it took about 10 minutes. January and February were still manageable with the life lab visit and classes. However, for the biopsy in March, I would have to go to the Grand River Hospital in Kitchener, which was 35 minutes away from where I lived. I did not drive, and the Uber fare to get there was very expensive, so I had to figure out an alternative.

I reached out to some friends, but they were not available. Finally, I took the courage to ask one of my housemates, with whom I was not close, but who had a car. He agreed, but I had to do his laundry as a way to thank him. He didn't ask for that. I just offered to help in return for his time. I went to the biopsy appointment on…and the procedure was quite simple – no pain, just minor discomfort. I did not know I would be sore, so I planned to go to class afterwards. I brought my bag, class materials, and everything. By the end of the procedure, I was sent to the recovery room, and that was when I realized I would not be able to make it to class. I emailed my professor right away, and she was understanding but mentioned that if I felt better, I could join the class late. I did not make it. The pain was strong enough that I could not walk properly, so I missed that one class. That was not the first time I missed class because of my health issues. That was just the beginning of the abruption to my studies because of kidney disease. I did not hear the biopsy results right away. It took the doctor a few weeks to get back to me. I kept going to classes as usual while waiting to hear the result. All these times, I was just fulfilling the duty of going to all the appointments, but I was not aware of how serious my conditions were. I was not too worried. I am not sure why I took it so lightly. Maybe it was because I did not have any major symptoms that affected my daily life, aside from sleepiness and tiredness. If I were to be sick and feeling unwell, I might have been more worried. I did not know then that kidney disease was fatal. I neither researched nor spoke to people. I just was not aware that it was serious.

I had the follow-up appointments a few weeks after, so I had to miss class and went to Kitchener again. Finally, the result came out, and I learned that my condition was caused by IGA and FSGS, which basically meant my immune system was attacking itself. That also means there was nothing the doctor could do to prevent it or stop it. The doctor in Grand River informed me that he would share my results with my nephrologist in Guelph, and that they would start treatment soon after my appointment. Unfortunately, I became ill before I could see my nephrologist. I was hospitalized twice and missed many classes.

More of the sickness and what went down in April and May will be detailed in the following chapter.

Chapter 10:

Getting Sick and Dialysis

I was not showing any symptoms of kidney disease until mid-April 2023. It was on the 14th of April, which was the New Year time in Cambodia, that I was hospitalized at the Guelph General Hospital. I had severe headaches and kept throwing up. I could not eat anything without vomiting, and I felt awful most of the time. The nurses gave me gravels for the vomit, but it didn't help. They gave me Tylenol for headaches, but it didn't work. I was in pain for most parts of the ten days at the hospital. My nephrologist came to visit me at the hospital and told me I had a kidney disease that was caused by an autoimmune disease (IgA and FSGS) and that I needed serious treatments. The issue was that the treatment could potentially trigger my manic episode. He was reluctant to implement the treatment and wanted to make sure I knew the implications. I was quite worried hearing that.

I couldn't risk getting manic, and I also knew I needed the treatment, so what do I do? I was discussing it with my mom, and we even thought about moving back to Cambodia, but later we realized we wouldn't be able to afford the treatment in Cambodia. Here in Canada, I have UHIP insurance that covers all treatment costs. Staying here makes more sense. Next, the decision was whether to take the treatment. After a long discussion with my mom and the doctor, we decided to risk having a manic episode as long as we get to treat the kidney disease. I had one more semester of school to finish, but with the risk of mania, I might not be able to work on my thesis and assignments properly. I was pondering this for almost a week about whether I could take on schoolwork during treatments. Finally, I decided to take a medical leave for the Summer and focused on getting better. It was a hard decision, but I am glad I made it. I was able to spend the time just taking care of myself and got much better. If I had dealt with schoolwork that Summer, I would have been stressed out and unable to take care of myself properly.

I took the treatment medication, but it didn't work well with me. By early May 2023, after taking a steroid (prednisone), I had a severe stomachache. I went to the ER again and stayed in the hospital for a week. The doctor had to end the treatment because it was working against my body. Now, the doctor had to figure out another treatment, which I didn't know was called dialysis. I didn't know I was reaching that stage. My nephrologist didn't tell me I was getting dialysis yet. He just made an appointment with me in two weeks and said to me that I would know the alternative treatment then. When I saw him again in mid-May, he told me I had reached the stage of receiving dialysis as my kidneys only functioned at 8%. Early in March, it was 33%. I had no idea how it went down so fast within the two-month time frame. I also started to develop other symptoms, such as swelling, when I was leaving the hospital the second time. My face, stomach, and feet were swollen. I could barely walk, or I'd get up once I sat down. My friend, Rez, told me I need to stop eating meat, and that was a big deal to me because meat was a big part of my diet. However, my dietitian didn't say anything about meat restrictions. She said I could still eat meat, but I needed to cut down my sodium intake.

After my appointment with the doctor, my mom had to leave for Hamilton, hoping to get some work on the farm. She was worried about me staying by myself, so we talked to one of my Cambodian friends, Sokhany, about the possibility of staying at her house. Sokhany was happy to hear that I wanted to come stay with her. She welcomed me with all her heart. Thus, the next two weeks before dialysis, I stayed at Shakespeare with her and her family. My symptoms were getting worse. My feet and stomach were swollen to an immense degree. My weight was around 60kg before, but by this time it had gone up to 80kg. I went to the ER at Stratford with Sokhany once when the swelling was too bad, and I had shortness of breath. The doctor prescribed Furosemide (water pills) to help with the swelling and sent us back home that night. That meant we didn't stay overnight at Stratford hospital. The rest of the time at Sokhany's was about reading, eating, and taking care of myself. My feet were so swollen that I couldn't wear socks by myself. Sokhany had to help me with that. She also got me some bigger clothes and a bag for my medicine. I was getting sad about my condition day by day as the dialysis was approaching, but I had no idea what dialysis was going to be like. They scheduled me for the 24th of May for a minor procedure to put a catheter in my chest for dialysis. On the 24th, Sokhna's mother-in-law, Kathy, took me to Grand River Hospital in Kitchener. Sokhany had to go to work, but she made sure to call and check in with me before the surgery. I was nervous, but her words calmed me down. I took the elevator to the 2nd floor for the surgery. As a nurse was showing the catheter, I was more scared to see a long pipe of plastic that was going to be attached to my body. Soon after, I was asked to go into the surgery room where I was introduced to the doctor who reassured me that the process wouldn't be long, and I wouldn't feel any pain as they would numb my skin before that. The doctor was right. I didn't feel any pain, and it went by so fast. After the surgery, I was sent to the recovery room for an hour before they sent me to the third floor for dialysis on that same day. Thus, the 24th of May 2023 marked my first day of dialysis. When I got to the dialysis room, a nurse asked me, "Are you scared?" I said, "Yes, I am." Then she was telling me that I shouldn't be, that there is no pain involved, and that I should just relax. She calmed me down and started the process of dialysis soon after. My first experience on dialysis started around 5 pm, and it was 3.5 hours. Turned out it wasn't so bad. There was no pain or discomfort, and I finished it with no complications. At 8:30 pm, it was done. Sokhany and her husband came to pick me up and asked how it went. I told them all was good. I was happy that all went well, so I was smiling when I saw them. There was only a slight discomfort from the catheter, but no major pain. I went back to their home that night and already felt a bit better, as the swelling had gone down.

I stayed with Sokhany and her family until the 29th of May, as I had to return to Guelph to pick up my husband. He finally got the visa and was scheduled to arrive on the 30th of May. I had done dialysis three times by then and looked much better (less swollen). I can't imagine what my husband would feel if he saw me before the dialysis. By the time I went to pick him up at the airport, I looked acceptable, not so sickly. I asked my friend, Le-Anne, and her husband for a favour: to pick up Promise at the airport, and they agreed. We waited about 2 hours before I got a call from Promise, who said he had landed. We took pictures and came home to let him rest. I thanked Le-Anne and her husband, and they said goodbye and left. I was extremely happy to see my husband, but I was feeling weak from dialysis, so that I couldn't show much excitement. I revealed the chest catheter to Promise, and he was shocked to see it. He had no idea my conditions were that bad. He later came to accept it and provided me with a lot of care.

We helped him get settled down and unpacked. The next day was my dialysis. I still had to go to Kitchener for the next two weeks. I was asking different friends for help taking me there, so arranging transportation was my main task. I left Promise alone at our rented house for the next few dialysis sessions. The week after, my doctor asked me to ask Promise to come to dialysis too because he wanted to talk to him and for Promise to ask any questions he had. Promise came and learned much more about my conditions from the doctor. One thing we learned was that I could not be pregnant any time soon due to my conditions. Promise accepted it and did not complain. I was glad to see that. I kept getting dialysis on Monday, Wednesday, and Friday for 3.5 hours for another week after that. Later, I requested to receive dialysis at Guelph instead, since it's closer to where I lived. They managed to find a spot for me in the second week of June, and I also applied for the Mobility bus to pick me up and drop me off each time for only $3 per trip. I continue to go to on dialysis three days a week for four hours each day, but I switched to Tuesday, Thursday, and Saturday. I feel weak after dialysis, but good on non-dialysis days. It went well for a while, but then I started having migraines and vomiting. One day, I vomited all over my shirt, and three nurses rushed to help clean me up. I felt so bad for them having to deal with my vomit, but I didn't mean to give them that trouble. Another time, I vomited in the Mobility bus on the way home. As for headaches, the nurses just gave me Tylenol, and sometimes it helped, sometimes it didn't. After the headaches and vomiting had happened several times, I decided to talk to the doctor to see if he could do anything to help. As a result, he made some changes to the dialysis machine, which indeed helped me with the vomiting and headache. After a week or two, I stopped vomiting and having headaches. I was thrilled.

Promise got a job on June 15th. He works five days a week and cooks for us on days off. I continued taking the mobility bus to the dialysis centre three times a week until July. Then the doctor reduced my dialysis frequency to two times a week, which was great. I only had to go in on Tuesday and Saturday, and I got to do other things on Thursday. My conditions remain stable for a while, and at the same time, I was doing some work-up tests for the transplant. I was hoping my oldest sister could donate a kidney to me, so I was working on her visa application as well.

Around August, the Doctor had recommended that I get a fistula on my left arm for dialysis instead of the catheter. He said it's safer, has a lower risk of infection, and that I can shower and swim. I agreed, and he made an appointment for me in September. On the 8th of September, I had the fistula surgery at the Grandriver hospital again. The procedure was painless. It was on my left wrist. I was put to sleep, and when I woke up, it was all finished. I didn't feel any pain. It took a while for the fistula to heal and be ready to use. I continued to use the chest catheter until January, when the fistula was ready. It was around the 15th of January when the nurse first started using my fistula for dialysis. It was painful because the needles were big (16 g), but it wasn't too bad, and it worked well the first couple of times. However, soon after, I had some health complications that put me in the hospital again, and the nurses stopped using the fistula for some time. More of the complication stories will appear in another chapter below. After the complications, I went back to doing dialysis three times a week because there was too much fluid to be taken out. So far, it is three times a week, and I have been doing well, except for occasional migraines.

Me at the dialysis center in the Guelph Satellite Unit! This was when I started using the fistula already.

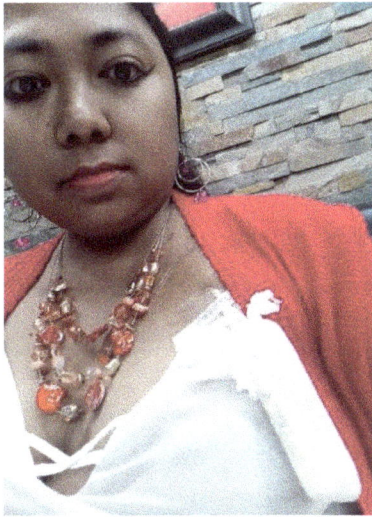

This was my chest catheter.

I don't have a picture in the hospital right after I got it. This was a while after.

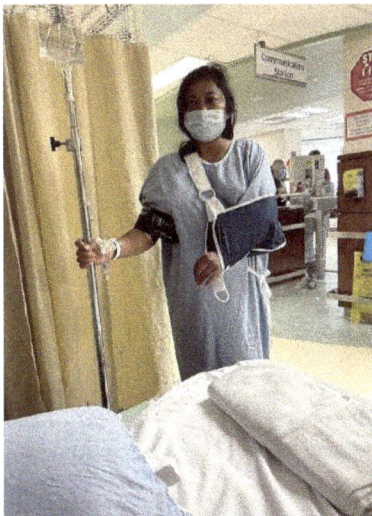

This was right after the fistula surgery. I stayed in the recovery room for a few hours and then I was discharged. I had this calf with me for a few days.

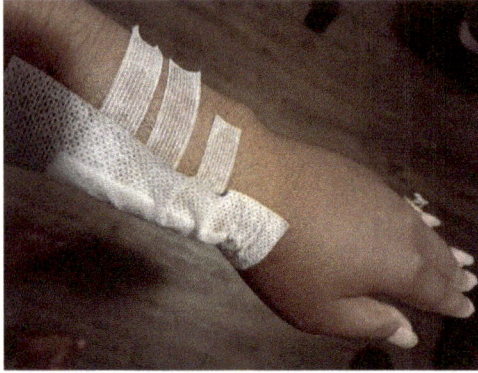

And these were the fistula when it was close to recovery. By now the pain was almost gone. It took a few more months after this until I started using it.

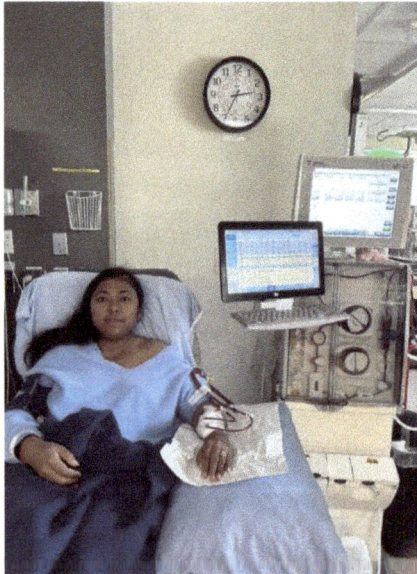

Me at the dialysis center in the Guelph Satellite Unit! This was when I started using the fistula already.

Chapter 11:

Fundraising and News about Transplant

Two months after being on dialysis, I had an idea of wanting to get a transplant in India. A lot of Cambodians back home choose this option as it is faster, and the surgery in Cambodia is more expensive and not as safe. I know a few people firsthand who have recommended that I go to India, as they had a great experience. They had their transplant surgery there, and now they are doing great, healthy, and happy. I wanted to be like them. I wanted to be healthy again, and Canada was not ready to provide the transplant. Their transplant program was too slow. I will have to go through a number of tests, and it takes a lot longer – it could be up to several years to get me on the transplant list and to finally get a kidney from a deceased person. Thus, I thought I could try to raise funds to get me to India for the transplant. In July 2023, I created a GoFundMe page to raise money for this purpose. I posted the fundraising advertisement on my social media, and the responses were beyond believable. I received a lot of support and love from old friends as well as people I didn't even know. I initially aimed to raise 40,000 CAD, but then I learned that it would not be enough to cover the costs of the transplant, dialysis, and the trip to India, so I increased my goal to 50,000 CAD. I received support bit by bit every day. I thought I could get to go to India with this money, but halfway through getting the money, my oldest sister, Chanrey, had a different idea. She said she wanted to get tested and see if she was a match and if she could come to donate for me in Canada. In return, she needed some of my fundraised money to pay off her loans and support her kids' education. I realized my money might be short for the trip to India, and I would have to work on getting the visa while traveling far away. It would be a lot of work and stressful, so I agreed to her suggestion to have her tested. It turned out that she had the same blood group, so that was a good start. She decided to come forward and email the transplant team in London, Ontario, about her intention and willingness to donate. She filled out some forms and had interviews with the team. The whole process took some time, and by the time she heard back their decision, it was in May 2024. They had told her that she could not donate because she had a serious kidney stone issue that kept recurring. Donating one of her kidneys could mean putting her at risk of getting a kidney disease in the future, which could be bad for her life. We had hope that she would be able to come to Canada for the surgery. We worked on her visa and even bought her a flight ticket, only to be disappointed by the news. By that time, I had already spent a significant portion of the fundraised money on her, so it was too late to save up for India. I was heartbroken and did not know what to do. I have two more sisters, but one is pregnant. I reached out to my younger sister, SereyRath, and asked her if she wanted to get tested. She did and found out her blood group was B+. Mine is O+. That means she cannot directly donate her kidney to me. She can still participate in the paired exchange program, where she donates to someone in the pool, and someone else from the pool will donate to me. At least, that was what we were told in the beginning. Thus, I requested my sister to get in touch with the transplant team in London and fill out questionnaires about her health. It took a few weeks for them to respond after she submitted the questionnaires and her blood group report, allowing the team to schedule an interview with her. Initially, they had planned to call her over the phone. However, when they called, without any clear reason, it kept going to voicemail. SereyRath was waiting for the call all day but heard no ringtone whatsoever. They then emailed her to reschedule, and this time, they said they would call through Webex. I was worried SereyRath might not know how to handle that kind of platform, but she surprised me. She managed to get connected when I tested out with her before the appointment. The day arrived, and she spoke with the team for nearly an hour, with a Khmer Translator assisting the conversation. After talking to them, she called me and told me her case was complicated. Because she lives so far away, she would not be eligible for the typical pair exchange program. Even if she donated, I would still not consider a living donor. Instead, I will still have to wait for a deceased donor, and it would still take at least one more year. SereyRath told me that the transplant team wanted to talk to me in person to discuss more about our case so that I would be clear about the options. She was talking with them in late May, and I was scheduled to meet the team on June 06 in London. I was disappointed, but I thought I should keep my hope up until I get to talk to them later in June. When I finally got to talk to the team, I learned that my current rank on the recipient list is number 11, and if my sister donated, it would bump me up to number 5. That means I would get a kidney much sooner with my sister's help. However, since I would not get the kidney from a living donor right away, SereyRath said she did not want to donate anymore. I respected her choice, so now I was left with no potential living donor. The transplant team in London suggested that I advocate and look for a donor on my social media platforms and ask my husband and family to do the same. Immediately, I started posting about my plight and searching for a stranger donor on my Facebook, LinkedIn, and Instagram. Many of my friends shared the post, and finally, I heard from a friend of a friend who lives in America that he wanted to donate to me, and he had the same blood type as me. I was extremely happy to hear the news. I got in touch with John right away, and we have been checking in with each other ever since. Just like the process that my sisters went through, John went through it the same things. He filled out the questionnaires, and he has been waiting for them to schedule an interview with him. It has been over three weeks since he submitted the document, but they have still not scheduled an interview with him yet. They are probably busy. Last time I chatted with John to ask about the update, he said they would call him back within 10 days. John has shown me incredible sympathy. He kept encouraging me to stay positive and wished that the process would be quicker for me. I cannot thank him enough for this amazing act of generosity, in which he was willing to donate one of his kidneys for me. More updates are on the way, and they will likely be included in my next book.

By the time I am writing this part of the book, it is August 2024, a year after I started raising money on GoFundMe. A year when I had no job and no income. Apart from supporting my sister/my family, I used the remaining money to support my living expenses. It has been an incredible help for me to survive and avoid getting too stressed. I cannot imagine how sad and stressed I would be without this money. The raised funds allowed me to live a good and positive life without the pressure to find work right away. I am forever grateful to all who have donated. It may not get to send me to India as hoped, but it helped me get to this stage where I have been fairly healthy and close to getting the transplant with John's generous act. Thank you so much to all who donated to my campaign and those who have shared it. Your money/generosity saved my life.

Chapter 12:

Wrapping up the degree while going for

dialysis

I had some personal and academic reason that made me switch from a PhD program to a master in the winter semester of 2023. By the end of Winter 2023 (when I found out I had kidney failure), I completed all courses for the Master's degree requirement except owing two assignments to my professors and the Major Research Paper. That means I would only need to be in school one more semester to complete all that. However, I was very sick, and with the doctor's concern that the treatment could trigger a manic episode, I was on the fan, not knowing if I could be in school full-time to complete the remaining work. I had dialysis three times a week, and I felt tired all the time. That alone concerned me that I would not be able to work.

Additionally, if mania did occur, I would be unable to work on the Major Research Paper or the ongoing assignment, and I would waste the tuition money. With that in mind, I decided I should take a semester off to focus on treatment and getting better. I filled out some paperwork to request for a semester off in the Summer and stayed home for the next four months to heal myself.

The Summer went by extremely fast. I kept going to dialysis, taking medication, and focusing on self-care. There were not many complications during these four months. In a blink, September arrived, and I had to reenroll in the program to complete the remaining requirements. In the first week of September, I worked on the two assignments that I owed to my professors from Winter 2023. I woke up in the morning, ate breakfast, and then started working on the assignment. By 12 pm, I headed to dialysis. When I returned at 5 pm, I cooked dinner, ate, and worked on the assignment again. It took me a bit over three weeks to complete the last two assignments. I submitted them and did not receive a grade until much later. By October, I found myself working on the Major Research Paper, following the same schedule of working on it in the morning and evening, while going for dialysis in the afternoon. It took a lot to focus on academic work when you were not feeling well. I was always tired, so I had to gather my energy properly before starting work. Sometimes, I had to eat a bit extra to ensure I had enough energy to focus on reading the materials and conducting the research. Some evenings, I could not work on the paper because I had migraines after dialysis, so I spent the evening resting. Some days, there were no migraines, but I just couldn't find the energy to wake up and work on the paper, so I slept all day long. There were just one or two days in a week that I was fairly productive. Due to my poor health, it took me nearly two months to complete the first draft of the Major Research Paper. I submitted the first draft and was waiting to get feedback from my advisor. It took her several weeks to respond with feedback. As soon as she got back to me, I reviewed the comments and started making the revisions. I took about two more weeks to finish my second draft. By the first week of December 2023, I received an email stating that my major research paper had been approved. I just got back from dialysis and felt lethargic, but the news brightened up my day. I was thrilled to have finally completed all the requirements for my third master's degree. I can now could rest properly without the academic stress. I told my husband the news, and he was very proud of me. The next day, we celebrated by going to eat at my favourite restaurant.

From then on, I went back to focusing solely on taking care of myself. My graduation ceremony is scheduled for June 2024. My next task was to search for a job. The search was super stressful and time-consuming. More on that will be shared in a separate chapter below.

Chapter 13:

More Health Complications

Dialysis kept going well for some time since the migraine and nausea stopped. I was doing well until February 2024. It was on the 13th of February, the day my mother was going to leave for Cambodia, that I started having complications again. My blood culture showed negative, meaning there was bacteria in my blood. I was at dialysis when the test came out. They had to let me finish dialysis first before they told me to go to the ER. I was supposed to take my mom to the airport after dialysis. The nurses insisted that I go straight to the ER. I wasn't sure what to do, but my mom's departure was a major event that I didn't want to miss. Thus, I refused to do what the nurses asked me to do, and I went to the airport with my mom. I was feeling unwell and thought I might have fainted along the way, but I made it to the airport safely. We dropped Mom off at the gate to the check-in area – we didn't go inside and left right after. The minute I got home, I called my husband to come take me to the hospital. He immediately got ready and came out to drive me to Guelph General Hospital. From where we parked to the ER room, it took about 6 minutes. I didn't make it to the ER properly because I was short of breath. My husband had to call for help, and a nurse gave me a wheelchair to sit on and proceed to get registered. I thought I was losing my mind, my life, I meant. I was struggling so badly with breathing that I felt I was not going to make it. My husband was just as scared. We got registered and waited for a few hours before we got to see the doctor.

After checking my blood work, getting an X-ray, and asking about my conditions, the doctor decided that I should stay in the hospital for a couple of days. A couple of days turned out to be a week. I was there from the 13th to the 20th. I spent my birthday (19th) in the hospital. They found out the next day that I had pneumonia on the right side of my lung, so I was getting antibiotics in the form of IV as well as medications. Since I was short of breath, I was also attached to an oxygen machine for most of my time there. At Guelph General Hospital, there is no dialysis machine.

There was something old-fashioned about the replacement dialysis machine, but it had to run for 7 to 8 hours. The regular dialysis machines run just half of that time. They didn't have a choice because Grandriver hospital was full, so they had to have me dialyzed with the replacement machine. I couldn't go to the bathroom for 8 hours, so a nurse was attending to my need to pee and pooping. I was first shy and embarrassed to ask from her about that, but after a few times, I got used to it. I was so grateful for the care I received. It was so attentive and caring. I didn't need to have my family member to take care of me as I would if I were to be in a Cambodian hospital. Despite the grave conditions of my health, I couldn't be more grateful that I am residing in Canada, a place with free health care. I would be struggling much more if I were to stay in my home country, Cambodia, financially and mentally.

On February 20th, I began to feel better, and the doctor decided to discharge me. I returned home and was doing okay for ten days, but then I got sick again on March 1st. This time, it was the left lung that had pneumonia. I was hospitalized again, but this time at Grandriver hospital in Kitchener because they have dialysis machines there. I stayed at Grandriver for 6th days. I was getting anti-biotics again as well as the oxygen. This time, I was getting dialysis as frequently as I needed. They just had to bring dialysis machine to my room on Tuesday, Thursday, and Saturday. After each time, they bring the machine back because it consumes a lot of space. Promise came to visit me every day after work. It was hard to drive at night, but he never complained. He would fall asleep while sitting next to me, and I would feel sad seeing that, but I loved to see him, so I didn't suggest for him to stop coming. The food was great, better than Guelph. They gave me sheets to choose the food that I preferred. The options were good and wide variety, so I enjoyed getting to choose each day. I was getting IV antibiotics as well as medication. I was getting better after the 6th of March, so they discharged me. I was thrilled to head home. For the next months to come, things were getting better. The 6th of March was my last day at the hospital for a while. I came back strong, and I continued to do well at dialysis since then except one incident in April where they could not find my vein and had to poke me five times. There was some bleeding, but it wasn't too bad. After that till as of today, there has been no complication with the fistula or dialysis again. I only hope it will stay that way. The only remaining problem is getting a headache/migraine during dialysis and after. My last episode at dialysis was on the 10th of October where the migraine was so bad I even vomited. It was awful. It had been a year since I stopped throwing out. I just hope that was the only time and that it will not happen anymore. We will have to wait and see. My nephrologist did make some changes on the dialysis machine, so there wasn't much else he could do. What he suggests for me to do now is to be pre-medicated. He wants me to take a 500 mg Tylenol 30 minutes before coming to the clinic. I tried, but it did not seem to help. I still got the headache regardless. I am going to talk to him again what else can be done. Other than the headache and occasional vomit, I am doing okay otherwise. The new focus for me at the moment is in job search and taking care of myself.

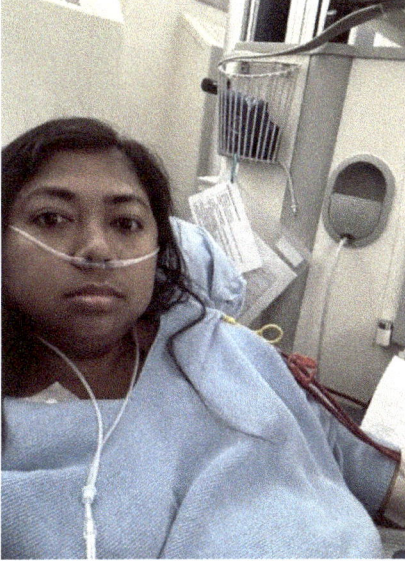
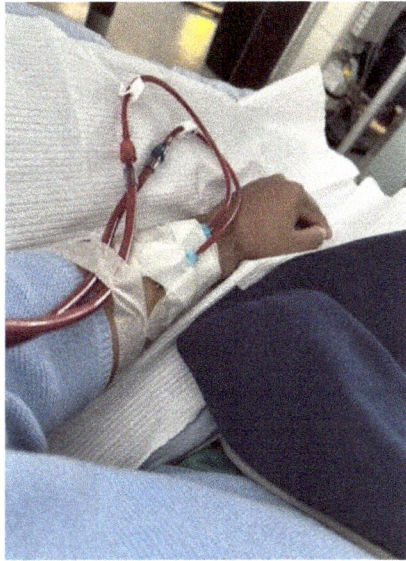

*A few of my pictures where I was getting dialysis and oxygen at the
same time because I was short of breath.*

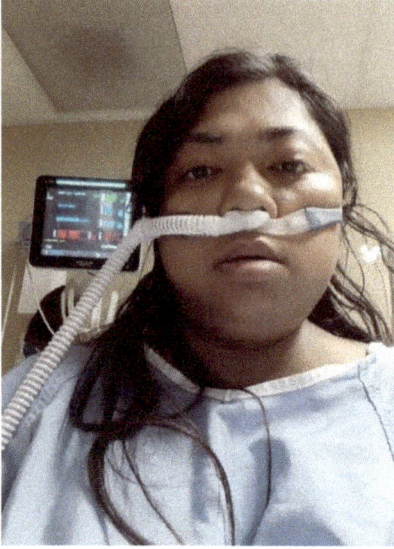

And this was when I had pneumonia the second time. They kept switching the tubes from the smaller one to the bigger one, depending on the severity of my shortness of breath.

Thanks to my friend, Sokhany, and her husband, Patrik, for the cake and for celebrating my birthday with me. Birthday: 19/02/2024

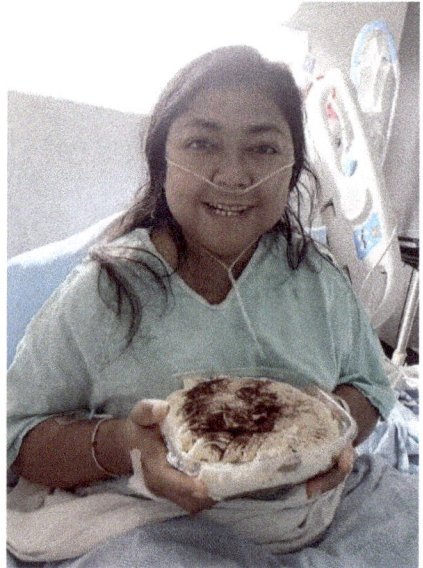

Chapter 14:

Job Hunt and Self-Care

The time went by so fast from the day I started dialysis to one year after. It went by in a blink. I finished all my schoolwork in December 2023, which was the 7th month I have been on dialysis. During these seven months, my life was consumed by dialysis and writing my thesis. By January 2024, when my thesis was completed, I shifted my focus to something else: the job hunt. I wrote and sent out hundreds of applications, the same resume, and different cover letters. Most of the jobs I applied to were research positions. I applied to different places, but most of them were in Toronto or Ontario. I had hoped I would get one in Toronto and move there with my husband. My mind was set on that dream. However, despite numerous applications, I kept receiving rejections or never hearing back from those employers. February came, then March, and April! I started getting really concerned that I would not find a job starting from May. That was when I began applying for other jobs, such as administrative positions and teaching assistant roles. I also tried out a few jobs at fast-food companies around Guelph. I thought it was time I took any job. I could not be picky anymore. I was desperate after submitting numerous applications over five months. None turned out positive. I kept applying, but I began to lose hope. I even attended a career fair in Kitchener with my husband on one weekend and submitted multiple copies of my resume there. Still, no good news appeared! By June, I finally got one interview. It was online, with a marketing company. I conducted the interview, and to my surprise, they interviewed all candidates simultaneously, asking just a few questions that barely allowed them to determine the qualifications. I didn't feel well after the interview, and as expected, I didn't get the job. My husband was very encouraging. He said, "It's okay. You'll try again in other places. Don't feel sad." I felt better after that, but still a bit disappointed.

I was always stressed during those intensive days of job applications, but I didn't forget to do something for myself. I made sure to get enough sleep and eat well. I also went for a walk regularly. I read and coloured picture books. Sometimes I meditate. I keep a journal with me where I write twice a week. I watched movies at night, mostly TV shows. My husband has different movie interests, so we don't often watch them together. We just hung out, cooking, talking, and spending time in downtown over the weekend. I had more free time than he did since he worked full-time, so I was often alone doing my own things. Applying for jobs at five to six places per day means spending 3 to 5 hours a day doing so. The rest of my time was for self-care (the activities I listed above) and dialysis. I didn't have time to feel sad about my life being dependent on a machine. It did not hit me hard until April 2024, when I received the news from my nephrologist that I could finally take out my chest catheter. That was the moment I felt more aware of my conditions and got a minute to reflect on my dialysis journey. It has been quite long and tiring so far. The news that I would be able to shower like regular people brought me so much joy that I couldn't wait for the removal day at the hospital. It has been 11 months since I have been on dialysis. I never complained a day for what I was going through until that day, 15th April, at the hospital, when I came to realize I was doing so well and was so accepting of my conditions and the hectic of having to go to the center doing dialysis twice or three times a week. When the doctor at Kitchener, Grandriver hospital, called my name for the removal procedure, I was reflecting on my journey, those 330 days where I had to cover my chest with a towel while taking a shower, had to sleep a certain way, and not be able to wear bras while always feeling something hanging and shifting down your chest. The fact that I knew my chest would be normal again and that I could shower properly made me ecstatic and super happy. As I walked into the procedure room, I was smiling hugely. I was unsure if the doctor and the team had seen that. The process took about 30 minutes. I did not feel any pain, just the pressure. In a blink, it was over. My chest was free after 11 months. Nothing made me happier.

I continued to apply for jobs until I received a response from Kelly Services, an interpreting company. It is a remote job where everything takes place on a computer. I took an entrance test, participated in a three-week training program, and passed a final test before being selected to work for them. I started the training on August 19th, 2024. That means it took me over six months to secure a proper job in Canada. I completed the training on September 11 and began taking calls immediately on the same day. I worked with Kelly until November 19, and then I transitioned to a new role with Certified Languages International (CLI), a US-based company that provides similar services. As I am writing this, it is my first day of work with CLI. I am not sure how well it will go, but it is a better-paid job with more opportunities to grow. I am hoping for the best in this role I am taking. I still have a big responsibility to support my family and fund my nieces' education. I need a well-paid job to be able to perform that role. Fingers crossed that all will go well with CLI.

Chapter 15:

Getting on the Transplant List and Transplant

Progress

Ever since I found out my kidneys were functioning at only 8%, I already knew I would need a transplant at some point. The question was when? Right after I started dialysis back in May 2023, I told my medical team upfront that I wanted to get tested for a transplant. They agreed and put my name in the list soon after. However, the process did not occur as quickly as I had hoped. It took them six months to get me to do the first screening tests of my heart and abdomen. It was in November. Before that, they did do my blood work once in every three months to see if I fit for a transplant, but I did not count that because blood work was just a preliminary process. Whether or not I would get to do a transplant would not depend on the bloodwork results alone. It would have to depend on several more tests. I was glad I was finally asked to get my heart and my abdomen checked in November. I thought all the other tests would be on the way too, but it wasn't until March of the following year that I was sent to do different tests, including an EKG and an ultrasound. Then I received the results, which showed that all tests were positive. I passed all the important stages to be eligible for the transplant except for the final evaluation at the University Hospital in London, where I will have my transplant. I was thrilled. I was getting closer to my dream. On May 17th, I received an email from the medical team in London asking me to come to the University Hospital for a two-day evaluation, where I will get the final word on whether I would be suitable for the transplant or not. The two days were scheduled for June 6th and June 11th. My appointment itinerary was as outlined below:

- June 06, 2024, at 8 am: Assessment bloodwork
- June 06, 2024, at 9 am: Meeting the social worker
- June 06, 2024, at 10:30: Meeting the transplant coordinator
- June 06, 2024, at 13:00: Outpatient preadmission
- June 06, 2024, at 15:30: Meeting with the surgeon
- June 11, 2024, at 13:00: Meeting the outpatient nephrologist

It was a full and busy day on the 6th. I was exhausted. My husband took me on the first day of assessment. On the second day, June 11th, Barbara took me because my husband was busy working. Since it was just one meeting on the second day, it was much more relaxing. After the two-day assessments, I gained a great deal of knowledge. I was a bit overwhelmed with all the information. I was also asked to complete two additional tasks: receive an MMR booster vaccination and visit the lab to take the QuantiFERON gold test.

Along with these two tasks, the transplant team also needed psychological clearance stating that I am fit for transplant, and the results from the renal biopsy that I did back in March 2023. I received the booster and had my blood work done the next day, but the reports from the biopsy and the psychology clearance took a while to be ready. It was not until July 27th that I received the activation letter, which finally put me on Ontario's Transplant Program waitlist, managed by the Trillium Gift of Life Network (TGLN).

It was such an exciting moment. From the first time I got dialysis to that moment, it took one year and two months. Just a few tests and blood work took me that long. The transplant team told me that with my blood type, I would have to wait for three to five years for a deceased donor. Taking one year to complete the transplant eligibility process is not a big deal, so I should be patient. However, when your life was dependent on a machine three times a week, four hours a day, and you get migraine and nausea so often, one year felt like forever. I was extremely happy to be on the waiting list at last. Now, I need to check with my living donor, John, about his progress. The donor team met with him in September 2024. He told me that everything went well and that he would need to meet with the social worker, complete two more tests, and undergo an ultrasound before they could confirm whether he is a match or not. When he told me this, I just had a severe migraine at dialysis, so it was a comfort knowing things were moving forward. Early in October, he had a meeting with the social worker, and he said it went well. Now, he just had to wait for the instructions on what tests he needed to do. For that, he had to wait three more weeks. They finally sent his doctor a letter instructing him to administer blood work to check the levels of electrolytes, creatinine, urea, hemoglobin A1C, and fasting glucose, as well as examine the 24-hour urine collection for protein and creatinine, perform a microscopic urinalysis, and test the urine for the albumin-to-creatinine ratio. Suppose the results are positive for the above tests. In that case, he will have to fly to London, Ontario, for an ultrasound that confirms the last criterion determining his suitability as a kidney donor. I am thrilled to hear about all this progress. In my head, I keep guessing the date when I will have the transplant. If the tests show concerns/problems and John cannot donate, my heart would be crushed. Dear God, let it all work out, and may I receive my new kidney from John; I beg of you. That was what I would go into in my prayers every night before I sleep.

John started doing the tests in early November. I look forward to hearing the results as I write this. The next day was Sunday. I was texting him to check when we could listen to the results. A few weeks passed, and I asked him for an update. He said his creatinine level was high. The team in London asked him to recheck the creatinine level and resend the result to him. This was in January 2025. In the meantime, on the 24th January at 12:15 am, I received a call from my hospital in London telling me that there was a kidney for me and that I should get to the hospital as soon as possible. However, I was the backup; there was no guarantee that I would get the kidney. There was one person who had priority over me.

Nevertheless, I should make my way there. I was beyond ecstatic. I called my husband and my mom to inform them of the good news while packing my bag. I finished packing in under an hour and thought I could get some rest. While trying to sleep, I got a call from the same number telling me that the kidney was no longer available. I dropped the phone on the floor, feeling completely let down. My excitement went to zero, and I wanted to cry. I did not cry, though. I told myself that at least now I know I'm at the top of the list.

The next day, I messaged John again about the update. He told me he would recheck the creatinine level soon and keep me posted.

A few months passed by, and it's April as of today when I am writing this. A few days ago, I messaged John asking for an update, and he said he had already sent the new result to the team in London. Now he's also waiting for the update.

I don't know if I will get John's kidney or a kidney from a deceased donor. All I know is that my time will be soon. I will be okay. My transplant will take place at any moment in the future. I need to be ready. This is what I keep telling myself.

Chapter 16:

Update on Transplant and Job

I t was on Tuesday night, 21st January 2025. I went to do dialysis as normal. Upon my return, when it was close to midnight, I got a call from an unknown number. I didn't want to pick it up because I thought it was a scam. They called again after about 5 minutes. This time, I picked it up. I did not know what to expect. I answered a call, and then a woman told me there was a kidney for me at the London Health Sciences Hospital. I was thrilled. I wanted to scream, only to hear further instructions that I was only a backup. There was someone in the line ahead of me, and if that person took it, I would be out of luck. But she wanted me to take the chance and come to the hospital by 3 am in the morning of the next day.

I agreed and started getting ready, and called Barbara to help with transportation. Promise was in Nigeria. Barbara was all I got. She was at the farm, so she arranged for Sovatana to bring me to the farm, and then she would take me from there to London. After the transportation was arranged, I called Promise and Mom to give the good news. They were extremely happy on my behalf, but they were sad they were not here with me. I finished the calls and waited for the time to come. Then, around 1:15 a.m., I received another call from the same number. I knew right away it was bad news. I picked up, and she told me the kidney was no longer available. My heart was broken. I thought it was finally my turn.

What the experience told me was that my turn is close. I am at the top of the list, and although I did not get it this time, it will happen in the near future. I should not lose faith. I am still waiting for that real call, and as I am writing this, it is the 15th of August 2025, seven months since that first call. I hope it is my turn soon, and I will not give up staying positive.

On the job front, I have applied for a new position in Canada, as my job with CLI is not going well. It is over the phone interpreting job, just like the job with CLI.

I arrived and had an orientation yesterday. The company is called CanTalk, a totally Canadian-owned company. I hope to start taking calls next Monday. Finger-crossed that it will go well, and I will get extra income to support myself.

Chapter 17:

Reality of Life after a Kidney Failure

Two things I experience after I found out I have kidney failure are – missing the old life and having to tolerate the unknown.

I miss the ability to drink as much fluids as I wanted. I miss the ability to eat any food I liked. I miss not having to rely so much on medication. I miss being able to urinate a lot and feeling light. I miss being able to go out and party on Thursday or Saturday nights. I miss being able to do different things and hang out with friends on Tuesdays, Thursdays, and Saturdays. I miss my old arm with no aneurysm. I miss the old face with no added fluids on. I miss looking good. I miss the old life so much I cry myself to sleep or in the shower. If it weren't for my therapists and support from my mom and my husband, I would have lost it.

The other thing I am experiencing is tolerating the unknown. I am talking about the transplant. For now, I do not know when that is going to happen. I keep going to dialysis three days a week hoping when I come back home, I would hear a call. However, it has been nearly a year since I got the back-up call early this year, and I still have not heard anything again. I have no clue when my turn will be, and tolerating this unknown has been one of the most challenging things in my life post kidney failure.

For you, other patients out there who are in the same boat, I feel you. I can relate to you, and I wish you nothing but all the best and that you will hear good news and receive a transplant soon. May we all recover at some point.

Finally, another thing about dialysis that affects me emotionally is the fact that I am almost always by myself during the dialysis treatments. For patients who have family in Canada, they often receive a visitor or visitors coming over to say hi and chat during treatments. Me, all I have is my husband! And he works 6 days a week, so he does not have free time to come say hi to me during treatment at all. It feels very lonely each time of the treatment and it would have been a lot different if I were to be sick in Cambodia where my family is. Lots of people would have come to visit me in each treatment. The only thing is that in Canada, I receive free treatments while in Cambodia I would have to pay. Thus, I guess the price I pay for that, which is being alone and lonely, is not too bad at all.

Chapter 18:

Promise and I

I do not have any relatives here in Canada. Promise is my only support that I can count on at any time. He is my best friend, my home, and my confidant. However, not surprisingly, my relationship with him is off and on. There are times when we fight, and there are times when we don't talk to each other. When that happens, I feel very sad. Because he is my only support, I feel lost when we do not get along.

In July 2025, we faced a significant issue that kept us apart for nearly two months. These two months were the longest months I have ever experienced. I missed him so much. Given my health status and my need to go for dialysis, not having him by my side were some of the most challenging times of my life. I realize at that time that Promise plays one of the most important roles in my life. I never want to fight with him again, and I never want to lose him. I hope that we will be together through thick and thin for the rest of our lives. The reason I am including this chapter is that I wanted to describe my life in a holistic manner, where not only my health is explained, but also my most important relationship here in Canada. As I deal with health challenges, Promise is the sole support that helps me fight through with hope and positivity. He cooks for me. He washed my hair when I had a catheter on my chest and could not wash my hair by myself. He takes to dialysis. He reminds me when to take my meds. He takes me to beautiful places. He is my personal photographer.

Most importantly, he is the first person I call when I want to share something with anyone. I love him to the bone. May our bond prevail and last forever.

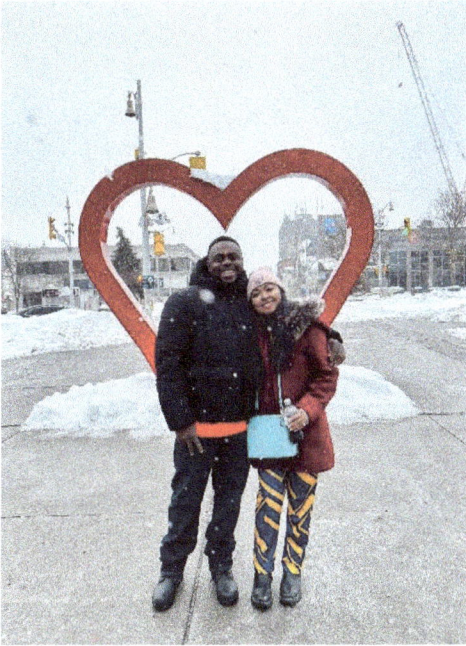

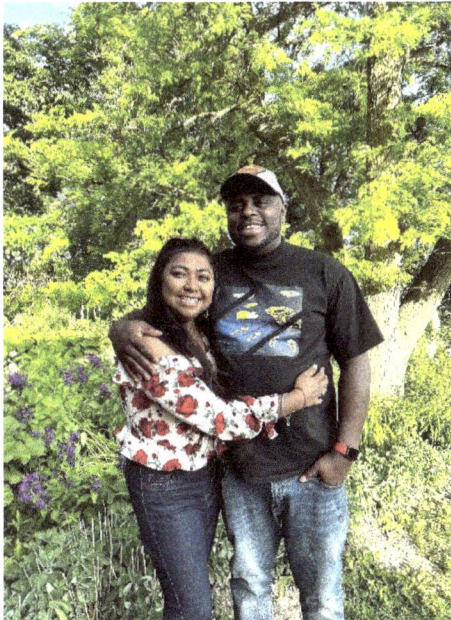

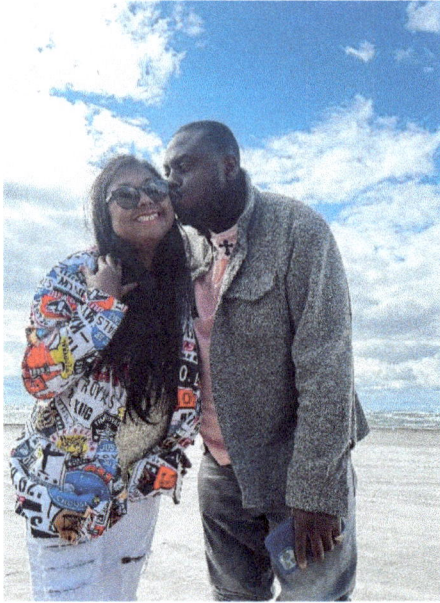

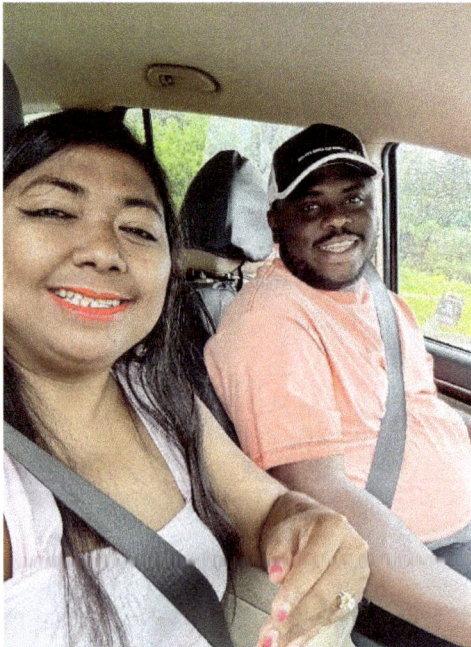

Chapter 19:

Tips on how to live with Bipolar

Medications play a huge role in keeping one stable with a bipolar diagnosis. I am a member of a Bipolar Support Group on Facebook, and learn that people are on a variety of meds. When I was first diagnosed back in 2017 and was hospitalized, I was put on Risperidone only. As I got better for a few months, my psychiatrist considered switching me to Depakote and Lamotrigine. Depakote did not work with me. Instead, it caused me to be more manic and even had several strange symptoms. When I took Depakote, I craved double or triple sounds playing at the same time. I would have a strong desire to play music while watching a movie or listen to two different types of music in two separate browsers. One sound system alone did not satisfy me. In addition, my appetite was over the roof. I ate like a starving person living under the Khmer Rouge area in Cambodia back in the 1970s.

After the Depakote try-out and failing, I was put back on Risperidone and kept going with Lamotrigine. You must have a knowledgeable psychiatrist who can work their magic, picking the right medication for you. Once they found the right fit of the meds for me, I was stable for another year. I chose to cut down the doses of Risperidone by myself when I returned to Cambodia, and that led to another psychotic episode. Same as the fourth episode in Canada. After that, I was taken off Risperidone and was put on Invega (the pills for the first few months and then the injection – once a month). I received the injection for over a year and then switched back to the pills. Later, when I was concerned and noticed feeling closer to depression, I was put on the second med, known as Lurasidone. These meds kept me stable for a good period of time, and these are some tips for people with bipolar:

- Help your psychiatrist figure out the right medications for you by carefully and accurately reporting your symptoms, and then keep track of the effects of the meds during the first try and the second try.
- Make sure to let the psychiatrist know what works and what does not. Switch to a different medication if necessary.
- Once you find the right medication, continue taking it regularly and do not miss any doses.
- Do not reduce the dose or stop taking the meds without consulting with your doctor/psychiatrist.
- Get enough sleep and eat healthy meals.
- Invest in a therapist. Having somebody to talk to lessens the burden on your heart and mind, thus relieving stress on yourself.
- Identify your triggers and avoid them whenever possible.
- Keep track of your progress and watch for changes in your behaviors/feelings. Notice and be mindful of any symptoms or changes in yourself and your mental state. Report those to your psychiatrist as soon as possible so that necessary steps can be taken, including adjusting the meds.

It is not a life anyone desires to have for people with bipolar, but those tips above would be helpful to help you navigate this new journey you may end up getting. There is no cure for people with a mental illness, but you can follow these steps to make sure your life is not too disastrous. I have had bipolar disorder for seven years, and I still manage to work full-time jobs, and obtain several postgraduate degrees, and live a happy life. I only had one episode of depression in late 2017 and early 2018; that was it. I have been able to stay away from depression since then, and it is 2024 now. My challenge is fighting psychotic episodes. I have had four major psychoses and ended up in the hospital twice. I have been stable since 2021, and I only hope it remains this way for a long time to come. Currently, I am continuing to take Invega (3mg) once every other day and Lurasidone (20mg) once per day. This combination seems to work quite well for me. I am feeling good and happy for the most part. Achieving three years of stability is not easy. I would say I am quite fortunate, and the credit goes to my amazing care providers at the Canada Mental Health Association (CMHA). I do not know what I would have done without them. Thank you, Dr. Muir, Drew, Anita, Karen, Stephanie, and Maegan, for your amazing support with my mental health. I owe you guys immense gratitude.

Chapter 20:

Tips on how to live with a kidney disease

Unlike a mental health disorder, a physical sickness requires more practical treatments, and once a chronic disease happens to you, you have to live with it every day. Bipolar for me is not an everyday thing. Symptoms come and go, and there are times I feel completely normal. Being a kidney patient, however, is a daily struggle. I get reminded that I have the disease every single day with my fatigue, sleepiness, and shortness of breath. I also cannot eat many different kinds of food, which I did not face when I only had bipolar. Moreover, I take more meds than I do for Bipolar. There is no cure/meds for kidney failure, but I take the medications for related conditions caused by the kidney not working. Most kidney patients have high blood pressure. I am one of them. Thus, I used to take eight pills just for controlling my blood pressure – 800mg of Labetalol (4 pills) and 120mg of Adalat (4pills). After a while, my blood pressure was still high, so my nephrologist increased it to 900mg of Labetalol (5 pills). On non-dialysis days, I also take water pills (Furosemide) to help me pee more. Those were another four pills (160mg). With Vitamin D in the morning, non-dialysis days meant taking thirteen pills at a time. That is just for the mornings. In the evening, I took around seven more for half the week, and six for the other half. The reason is that I take Invega (for psychosis) every other day, not daily. Another bipolar med is Latuda for preventing depression. The big junk is the same four pills of Labetalol, and finally a pill of Replavite (Vitamin B & C). Total, I took up to twenty pills per day. It sounds like a lot because it is. I resented getting up and taking 13 pills, but I did not mind nine pills that much. After my school insurance ended in August 2024, my doctor made some adjustments to my blood pressure pills because the costs for Labetalol and Adalat were too much to manage. Instead of taking five pills of Labetalol twice per day, I now take just one pill of Bisoprolol (10mg) once per day before bedtime. Instead of 4 pills of Adalat, I now take one pill (10mg) of Amlodipine in the morning only. Besides staying on top of taking medications, here are some suggestions for kidney patients to take care of themselves:

- Eat a balanced meal three times a week, consisting of enough protein, calories, fruits, and vegetables.
- Cut down on salt as much as you can
- Limit potassium and phosphorus intakes to as minimal as possible
- Exercise (just go for a walk or stretch if you can't do heavy work) and implement self-care activities
- Have your labs monitored routinely as recommended by your kidney specialist
- Know your hemoglobin level
- Communicate any symptoms – new or worsening. Don't just assume that they are "normal" or related to another problem.
- Understand the benefits and risks of all treatments
- Keep follow-up appointments and take medications as prescribed
- Continue getting dialysis and do not miss it (missing two weeks means death)
- Participate in support groups (online and offline) and keep learning about the kidney disease as much as you can

For those who have a fistula, a few additional steps to take are as follow:

- Take care of the fistula by keeping it clean and dry

- Do not carry/lift heavy things with the arm that has the fistula
- Request the nurses to poke at different spots on the fistula to ensure one spot is not overly swollen
- If a hematoma occurs, make sure to ice it
- When you're hooked to the machine, make sure you do not move that arm

If you can follow most or all of the above tips and tricks, you will be more likely to stay alive for a longer period and suffer less. Life with a kidney disease will not be able to go back to the same as before, but the tips above will help you able to tolerate this illness better and smoothly. You will not be cured, but you will not feel too sick or awful. However, there are cases where you follow all these steps, and you still struggle with unpredictable complications. For instance, I still have migraines and vomiting occasionally at dialysis. My nephrologist has not yet been able to eliminate it completely. Plus, I also had pneumonia twice. Some other patients had other issues such as migraines, restless legs, blood clots, and others. It is also challenging to maintain a low creatinine level and a high eGFR level. I fail at these two numbers. My creatinine keeps on increasing. It is at over 1100 for my last lab result in early October. My eGFR is 4, the lowest was 3. I am at a loss for how to improve these two numbers, but at the same time, my nephrologist reminds me that I am still okay. Those numbers tend to be like this for dialysis patients. What I can control well is my potassium and my phosphorus. I have been good with them. My hemoglobin level is also good. I receive iron supplements once a month, and they have been sufficient as well. I go for a walk almost every day, and I also enjoy swimming, yoga, and cycling at the YMCA. I also meditate sometimes, which often helps with both my mental and physical health. I hope you find some of these tips helpful; the overall tips for living a better life while facing health challenges will be discussed in the next chapter below.

Chapter 21:

Tips on how to endure life adversity and health challenges

Before I found out I had bipolar disorder and renal failure, I also went through a lot of hardship, especially before I went to college. I helped my mom earn money since I was eight; I travelled to sell food/grilled chicken on bumpy and muddy roads; and I got only a few hours of sleep some nights. I thought my life was pitiful. I often felt sad about myself and angry with life. What kept me going was the fruit of education. I told myself that things would be better once I got my higher education and a good, well-paid job afterward. As predicted, my life improved significantly when I attended college and pursued my master's studies. Little did I know I would be confronted with a new challenge, this time medical and incurable.

When I got diagnosed with bipolar, I was manic and did not understand the implications until the weeks after I was discharged from the hospital. I knew my life was not going to be the same, but nothing prepared me for what was coming next: the depressive episode. It was the most dreadful experience in my life. I thought I had known depression, but I was wrong. Before, it was just a simple sadness. Clinical depression, on the other hand, exhausts you. It makes you feel utterly worthless and low. You just don't want to do anything besides sleep. You don't want to eat, and you don't want to shower or clean yourself. You do not enjoy anything you spend time on, and the worst part is, you want to end everything. It was scary and morbid. Those who have never experienced it will never understand the depth of that awful feeling. I just hope that you and I will never have to go through that again. What got me through the depression was the medication and the support from my family and friends. Therapy also helps.

Eating nutritious food, doing yoga and meditation, and other forms of exercise have also been proven to help with depression. Some people struggle with it for a long period of time, and it does not seem to have a cure, but my advice is to take the med and talk it out with close friends, family, and professionals. Staying alone and not sharing is most dangerous. Seek help from various people as much as you can. If the stress involves money, it gets trickier. It may require support beyond friends and family, including the government or loan providers. As long as you talk to people for support and resources, there should be a way out.

For psychosis or a manic episode, it is harder to predict or prevent it because it is sudden and random. There may be signs/symptoms to take notes of, but sometimes there aren't. Some tips and tricks for maintaining a little control over preventing it include taking medications regularly, getting enough sleep, eating healthy foods, engaging in exercise and self-care, and avoiding triggers such as stress, a stimulating environment, and substance use. Major life changes such as divorce or job loss can also trigger mania. When these changes occur, be sure to take preventive actions and start reaching out to your therapist/psychiatrist to get help in advance. When you do see symptoms of a manic episode, check into the mental health center as soon as you can, and do not worry about everything else at home. Your health, including mental health, is your top priority. Do not feel guilty for leaving everything behind. Once you are okay, you can take care of those. Just not then when you are sick or not well.

Living with a physical illness, including kidney failure, requires a lot more work. I was reading a book about a woman who has an autoimmune disease that the doctors do not fully diagnose, and she is extremely stressed about it because she wonders what the causes are. If you know the causes of your illness, you are one step ahead of most people. The next step is to work with your doctor to determine the cure or treatment. If you have cancer, chances are you will never be cured and you will end up being dead in a couple of years. That has to be the most dreadful disease that I do not know how other patients, or I, can help advise. However, if you are a kidney patient like me, the tips and tricks in chapter 18 will help you navigate through this challenging experience. In addition to those tips, it is essential to remain as positive as possible. That is extremely pivotal. Once you find out your kidneys are failing and when you feel tired all the time, you could lose hope and become utterly depressed if you do not watch yourself. You must remain optimistic to combat this disease. If you can maintain a good attitude toward it and do not give in to depression, you will tend to be doing much better and live an okay life. You might not be happy all the time, but you will have the strength to go on taking medications daily and enjoy some fun times with family, friends, and loved ones.

No matter what sickness you have, physical or mental, the two things you need before anything else are the medications from professional doctors and support from loved ones. Be sure you will not hide your illness/problem and try to solve it all alone. You must seek help and support from those around you. Also, it is essential to take it one day at a time and not worry too much about what will happen in the future. Live in the present and try to stay positive. Continue taking your medication, eat a healthy diet, get enough sleep, exercise regularly, and practice self-care. It is hard, but it is not impossible to live with chronic diseases or mental disorders. I live with them and survive. You can too.

Chapter 22:

Reflection and What Now?

It is essential to acknowledge that despite my new health challenges, I was able to earn another higher degree in a different country and secure a few new jobs, as well as complete this second book. In this manner, I hope I have shown the audience how I beat the odds, which is the title of the book. So, what now? Where am I at?

As I write this on September 12, 2025, Promise and I are back together, and we are doing much better. I also hope that I get a real call for a transplant as soon as possible. I am still doing dialysis three times a week, and my health is stable for now. I now hold three master's degrees and one bachelor's degree. Once I receive my transplant, I will consider pursuing a PhD or enrolling in a practical course/training program to acquire a new skill, such as Early Childhood education or nursing. I will need to consult with a few people to help me make that decision. I am also writing my third book, which tells the story of my mother's life and how her strengths continue to inspire me to this day. Professionally, I continue to work as an interpreter for both CLI and CanTalk. I will continue doing this for as long as my physical abilities allow.

I have applied for permanent residency in Canada, but we won't know the decision until a year or a year and a half from now.

I still miss my father a lot, and to remember him, I am going to get a tattoo reminding me of our time together. I am still deciding what exactly I should get, but I have a few ideas and will finalize it shortly. Maybe I will include the picture of the tattoo in my next book.

That's it about my life right now. I am not sure where life will take me. If it is going to be Canada permanently or somewhere else. Let's see, and adios for now.

Some of my pictures from the graduation day:

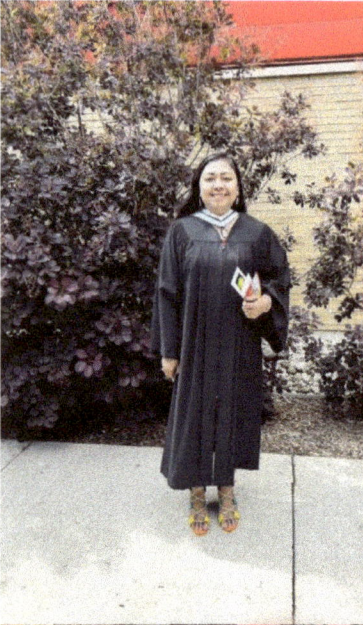
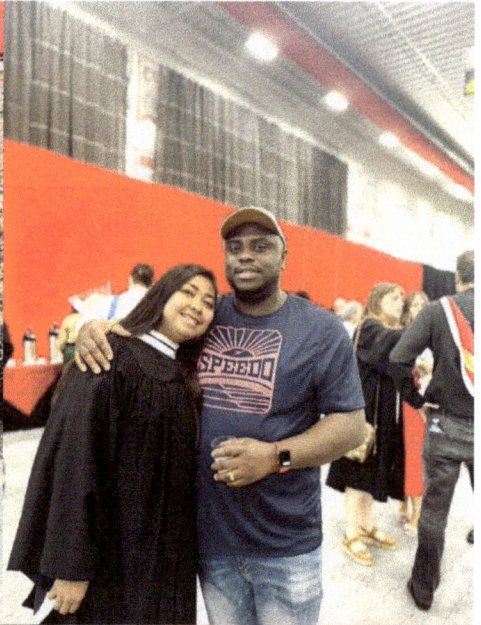
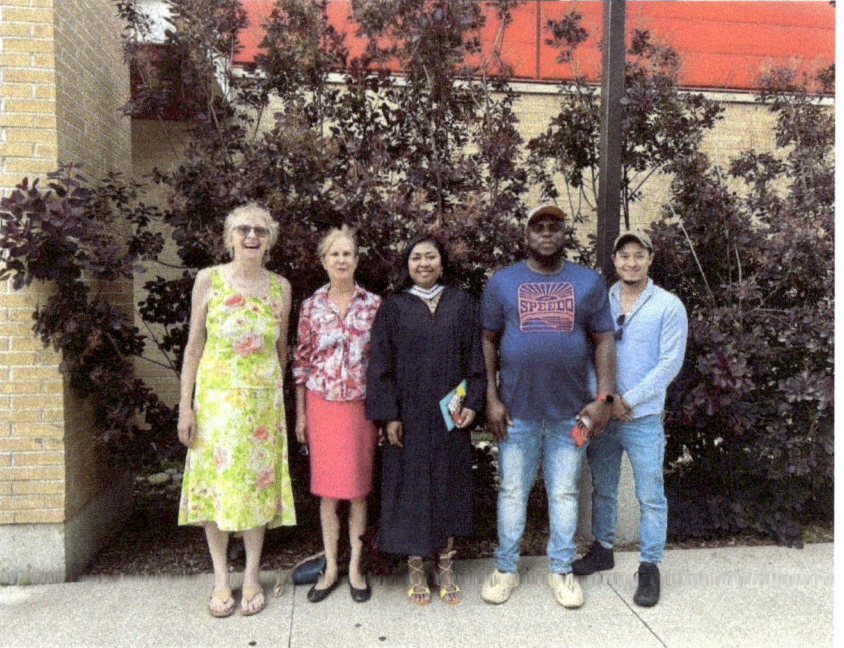

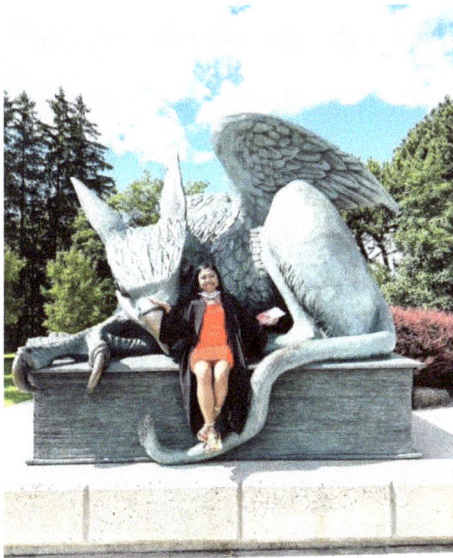

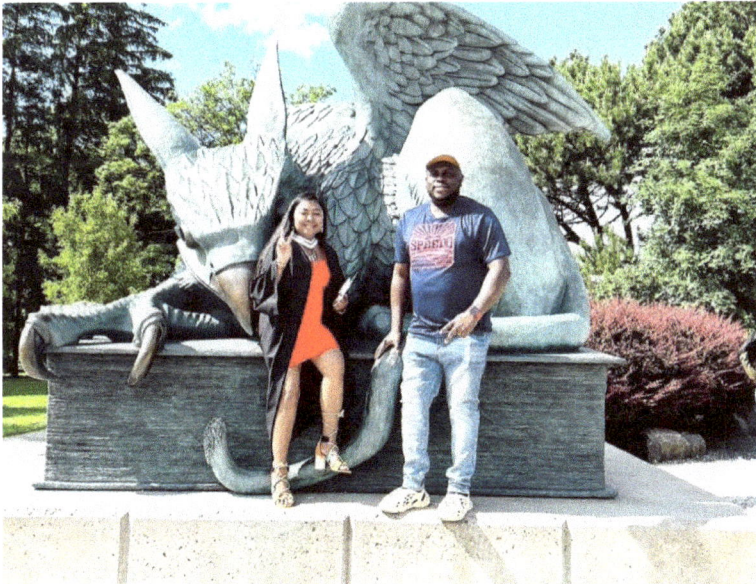

About the Author

Saren Keang was born and raised in a small village in Siem Reap, Cambodia. She holds a bachelor's degree in Asian studies from Asian Universities for Women, Bangladesh, and three Master's degrees in Sustainable International Development and Conflict Resolution and Coexistence from Brandeis University, USA and in Sociology from the University of Guelph, Canada.

She's an advocate for women's rights and gender equality and has spoken publicly about this issue in Cambodia, Bangladesh, Thailand, and the USA. She's also a co-founder of Dare and Dream, an aspiring social enterprise that aims to empower Cambodian rural female students through mentorship programs.

Saren is the author of two books, "A Long Way from Home" and this one: "Beating the Odds," as well as an Oral History Manuscript called "Life Under the Khmer Rouge: An Oral History on the Survivors of the Cambodian Genocide".

Today, Saren lives with her husband, Promise, in Guelph, Canada. In her free time, Saren enjoys reading, writing, photography, practicing yoga, and playing badminton.

Follow her here:

Facebook: Keang Saren - កាំងសារ៉ែន
Instagram: Saren Keang

Contact Details:

Email: keangsaren@gmail.com
Telephone: +1 519 760 0875

www.ingramcontent.com/pod-product-compliance
Lightning Source LLC
Chambersburg PA
CBHW052118030426
42335CB00025B/3037